'Raluca Soreanu has become an indispensable thinker in contemporary psychoanalysis. With dazzling precision, she shows that the psyche's fragments are not detritus but lively actors in trauma, memory, and repair. This book outlines a "minor psychoanalysis" of scars, organs, catastrophe – an audacious re-staging of Ferenczi that re-opens psychoanalysis to its most experimental, timely, and unruly possibilities.'

Patricia Gherovici, *Psychoanalyst and Author of* Transgender Psychoanalysis

'Soreanu's return to Ferenczi, like Lacan's return to Freud, levers us not into the past but a transformational future, a new psychoanalytic imaginary that is oblique, tentacular, visceral, surreal, decolonial. Here is a vocabulary of pliable elements, mimicry, asynchronous temporalities, fluid bodies, mosaics of dead and alive fragments – a psyche sensorially gripped and dismembered by the scars of time, but endowed with radically creative capacities and modes of registration and survival. Compelling, poetic, and precise, anchored throughout in luminous clinical narratives and a rigorous didactic concern with process, this is an epoch-making contribution to the emergent Ferenczian tradition: rerouting the mainstream into fascinating, life-preserving waters.'

Matt ffytche, *Professor of Psychoanalytic Studies, University of Essex, U.K. and Editor,* Psychoanalysis and History

'In her strikingly lyrical text, Raluca Soreanu elucidates what "being in fragments" might mean psychically. Drawing on the work of Sándor Ferenczi, Soreanu takes us beyond the static and repetitive temporalities of dissociation and splitting, and suggests that rather than the discarded elements of trauma, psychic fragments have a life of their own. Through clinical vignettes she shows us how patient and analyst can create a montage of such fragments, producing transformations in suffering through the co-creation of new and surprising forms of psychic life. Breathtakingly original, Soreanu offers us an entirely new thesis on trauma.'

Lisa Baraitser, *Psychoanalyst and Professor of Psychosocial Theory, Birkbeck, University of London, U.K.*

The Psychic Life of Fragments

The Psychic Life of Fragments rethinks trauma and psychic fragmentation starting from the psychoanalytic clinic.

What does it mean to work with fragments in psychoanalysis? What is the psychic life of fragments? And what can a fragment do? Raluca Soreanu writes about trauma, fragmentation and the radical plasticity of the psyche. Reconstructing Sándor Ferenczi's trauma theory, she articulates an original vocabulary of fractures, splits, atomisations, pulverisations, leakages, detritus and psychic de-materialisation along with new formations, protective membranes, expansions, contagions and growths. She approaches the scene of trauma from new angles, paying attention to oblique lines and asymmetric encounters. Mobilising clinical and literary vignettes, this book further argues for a minor psychoanalysis, one that emerges at the intersection of four types of theoretical-clinical experimentation: a psychoanalysis of scars, a psychoanalysis of organs, an eventful psychoanalysis and a blue psychoanalysis.

This book is important for clinicians and trainees in psychoanalysis, for mental health practitioners working with trauma, and for psychosocial and psychoanalytic thinkers. It is written to be used, between the psychoanalytic chair and the couch, especially at challenging times, in the transference and in the world.

Raluca Soreanu is a psychoanalyst and professor of psychoanalytic studies in the Department of Psychosocial and Psychoanalytic Studies, University of Essex, U.K. She is a member of the Círculo Psicanalítico do Rio de Janeiro, Brazil, and of the Site for Contemporary Psychoanalysis, U.K.

RELATIONAL PERSPECTIVES BOOK SERIES
ADRIENNE HARRIS & EYAL ROZMARIN
Series Editors

STEPHEN MITCHELL
Founding Editor

LEWIS ARON
Editor Emeritus

The Relational Perspectives Book Series (RPBS) publishes books that grow out of or contribute to the relational tradition in contemporary psychoanalysis. The term *relational psychoanalysis* was first used by Greenberg and Mitchell to bridge the traditions of interpersonal relations, as developed within interpersonal psychoanalysis and object relations, as developed within contemporary British theory. But, under the seminal work of the late Stephen A. Mitchell, the term *relational psychoanalysis* grew and began to accrue to itself many other influences and developments. Various tributaries – interpersonal psychoanalysis, object relations theory, self psychology, empirical infancy research, feminism, queer theory, sociocultural studies and elements of contemporary Freudian and Kleinian thought – flow into this tradition, which understands relational configurations between self and others, both real and fantasied, as the primary subject of psychoanalytic investigation.

We refer to the relational tradition, rather than to a relational school, to highlight that we are identifying a trend, a tendency within contemporary psychoanalysis, not a more formally organized or coherent school or system of beliefs. Our use of the term *relational* signifies a dimension of theory and practice that has become salient across the wide spectrum of contemporary psychoanalysis. Now under the editorial supervision of Adrienne Harris and Eyal Rozmarin, the Relational Perspectives Book Series originated in 1990 under the editorial eye of the late Stephen A. Mitchell. Mitchell was the most prolific and influential of the originators of the relational tradition. Committed to dialogue among psychoanalysts, he abhorred the authoritarianism that dictated adherence to a rigid set of beliefs or technical restrictions. He championed open discussion, comparative and integrative approaches, and promoted new voices across the generations. Mitchell was later joined by the late Lewis Aron, also a visionary and influential writer, teacher and leading thinker in relational psychoanalysis.

Included in the Relational Perspectives Book Series are authors and works that come from within the relational tradition, those that extend and develop that tradition, and works that critique relational approaches or compare and contrast them with alternative points of view. The series includes our most distinguished senior psychoanalysts, along with younger contributors who bring fresh vision. Our aim is to enable a deepening of relational thinking while reaching across disciplinary and social boundaries in order to foster an inclusive and international literature.

A full list of titles in this series is available at https://www.routledge.com/Relational-Perspectives-Book-Series/book-series/LEARPBS.

Notes

1 Greenberg, J., & Mitchell, S. (1983). *Object Relations in Psychoanalytic Theory.* Cambridge, MA: Harvard University Press.

The Psychic Life of Fragments

On Splitting and the Experience of Time in Psychoanalysis

Raluca Soreanu

Routledge
Taylor & Francis Group
LONDON AND NEW YORK

Designed cover image: Hannah Höch, *Aus der Sammlung: Aus einem ethnographischen Museum* [*From the collection: From an ethnographical museum*] 1929

First published 2026
by Routledge
4 Park Square, Milton Park, Abingdon, Oxon OX14 4RN

605 Third Avenue, New York, NY 10158
and by Routledge

Routledge is an imprint of the Taylor & Francis Group, an informa business

British Library Cataloguing-in-Publication Data
A catalogue record for this book is available from the British Library

ISBN: 9781032715919 (hbk)
ISBN: 9781032715896 (pbk)
ISBN: 9781032715926 (ebk)

DOI: 10.4324/9781032715926

Typeset in Times New Roman
by Deanta Global Publishing Services, Chennai, India

For Lorna

Contents

Figures

Acknowledgements

I am grateful to Jenny Willner and Jakob Staberg for many precious and enlivening conversations, for the time we gave each other, and the things we made together over the past five years. I am also grateful to Monika Perenyei for the fresh and energising exchanges and for opening new avenues of thought for me. I am indebted to Matt ffytche for being a generous reader and an inspiring and brilliant interlocutor. I thank Irina Culic for the enabling care for my text and its process, and for the constant support, in times luminous and dark. A special thank you to Erzsebet Strausz for her transformative effect on the process of writing and for allowing new lighter explorations to take shape in the year I completed this book. I am grateful to Lisa Baraitser for her enduring, rich and thoughtful presence over the past decade.

I am deeply grateful to the FREEPSY research collective. Their inspired and dedicated work has been part of my day-to-day over the past three-years, as I shaped the manuscript into its current form: Ana Čvorović, Ana Minozzo, Ana Tomcic, Ewan O'Neill, Ivan Ward, Julianna Pusztai, Lizaveta van Munsteren and Sarah Keeling-Smith. I also thank FREEPSY fellow-travellers Andréa Guerra, Felicity Callard, Gabriel Tupinambá, Harriet Mossop, Joanna Ryan, Magda Schmukalla, Patricia Gherovici and Susana Caló.

Thanks to the 'Waiting Times' research team for their input in thinking through matters of time and temporality: Lisa Baraitser, Laura Salisbury, Jocelyn Catty, Michael Flexer, Martin O'Brien, Deborah Robinson, Stephanie Davies, Kelechi Anucha and Martin Moore.

I am thankful to my colleagues in the Department of Psychosocial and Psychoanalytic Studies at the University of Essex in the U.K. for creating an excellent and anchoring environment for thinking and writing. I thank my psychoanalytic society, Círculo Psicanalítico do Rio de Janeiro in Brazil, for being an important place of return. Thanks to Claudia Garcia, Carlos Lannes and Carla Penna. Thank you also to Marina Ribeiro and Daniel Kupermann. I am grateful to the members of the social clinic Instituto de Estudos da Complexidade in Rio de Janeiro for being a deeply transformative clinical collective. A special thank you to Tereza Estarque and Fatima Lobo Amin.

Thanks to the many psychoanalysts and thinkers who have shared their insights on the work of Sándor Ferenczi with me and who have responded to my work, especially Antal Bókay, Jay Frankel, Giselle Galdi, Adrienne Harris, Galina Hristeva, Endre Koritar and Judit Szekacs. In the past 13 years, I have presented parts of this manuscript to numerous congresses, conferences, workshops, and clinical encounters, in a plural and beautiful process of crystallising the book into its current shape – for each of these occasions, I am deeply grateful to the organisers, the audiences, the co-panellists and discussants. I have also had the opportunity to teach on and around the work of Ferenczi at psychoanalytic societies, at the Freud Museum London and at universities around the world. The brilliant questions my students and trainees asked prompted new thoughts, for which I am grateful. A special thank you to the students of the MA in Psychoanalytic Studies at the University of Essex in the U.K. I thank my clinical supervisees, who enrich my clinical thinking every week. I thank my PhD students for the many inspiring exchanges which have sharpened my work. Thanks to Christine Taylor.

I thank Ana Maria Furtado: I hope this book can be the gift I promised.

I thank Adrienne Harris for being a brilliant interlocutor and editor and for welcoming the book to the series. I am also grateful to Steven Kuchuck for the editorial work. I thank Kate Hawes, Deepika Batra and Aakriti Aggarwal at Routledge for their work.

I am grateful to Agnes Meadows for the great care of my text and for her supporting presence. I thank Hannah Crago and Sean Andersson at the University of Essex for facilitating the publication of this book in Open Access form. Thanks to Hugo Coria for the very generous help with design matters.

The writing of Chapters 1 and 3 of this book was supported by a UKRI Frontier Research Grant ['FREEPSY: Free Clinics and a Psychoanalysis for the People: Progressive Histories, Collective Practices, Implications for our Times', EP/X022064/1]. The writing of Chapters 2 and 4 was supported by the Wellcome Trust ['Waiting Times', 205400/A/16/Z].

Earlier versions or sections of some chapters have appeared in journal article form. A part of Chapter 1 appeared as 'Soreanu, R., The Psychic Life of Fragments: Splitting from Ferenczi to Klein', *American Journal of Psychoanalysis*, 78(4): 421–444, 2018. It is reprinted by permission of the Editors and Palgrave Macmillan. Parts of Chapter 2 appeared as 'Soreanu, R., Something Was Lost in Freud's Beyond the Pleasure Principle: A Ferenczian Reading', *American Journal of Psychoanalysis*, 77(3): 223–238, 2017 (reprinted by permission of the Editors and Palgrave Macmillan); and 'Soreanu, R. The Time of Re-living: For an Eventful Psychoanalysis', *Vestigia*, 2(1): 132–153, 2019 (reprinted by permission of the Editors). A part of Chapter 4 appeared as 'Soreanu, R., Ferenczi's Times: The Tangent, the Segment, and the Meandering Line', *American Imago*, 73(1): 51–69, 2016. It is reprinted with permission of the Editors and Johns Hopkins University Press.

I thank Ethan for adding new colours and forms of joy to life. I am grateful to Lorna for the anchoring love, for her courageous and inspiring work, and for the beauty of the everyday. This book is dedicated to her.

Prelude

On Walking across a Mosaic

In one of our sessions, my patient Ava asked me: 'Do you know that painting by Dali? It's a Renaissance girl-head exploding?' And then she continued: 'That's how I feel, most of the time, in pieces and like all my organs are out of place…'. I did know the painting well, a reproduction of it was hanging on my wall in my youth. It is the 1951 work by Salvador Dali, 'Raphaelesque Head Exploding', which he created following the atomic bombing of Hiroshima in 1945. He painted a striking and delicate halo of the Madonna, exploded as a nuclear mushroom. When Ava brought it up, I instantly remembered a detail: among the many shapes, objects and part-objects it contained, within the cloud of disparate particles making up the head-figure, there was a strange form: a wheelbarrow. It sat somewhere along the line of the neck or the shoulder. I thought then of a psychic fragment that can help carry a big psychic weight of pain, or even the weight of the less-shaped fragments, which don't bear any resemblance to a familiar form. Just like one would carry sand in a wheelbarrow. By making this analogy, Ava helped me better accompany her state of being in fragments. She helped me further imagine it and ask new questions about her psychic fragmentation. This book continues in the space opened by this utterance by my patient Ava.

The pages opening before you, reader, are an exploration of the psychic life of fragments. I think about trauma and about the radical plasticity of the psyche, and I ask what we can do *with* trauma, in the psychoanalytic clinic, if we constantly work to enrich our clinical imagination around psychic fragmentation. This book is a montage, a particular arrangement of fragments of clinical encounters and of elements for a psychoanalytic theory of fragments. By working with the fragments, I show that trauma is not a still

DOI: 10.4324/9781032715926-1

space ruled by the death drive, placed outside of meaning and symbol, but also ego-constructive and memory-constructive.

The clinic of our times is traversed by references to a range of 'dissociative' processes and to forms of psychic splitting and fragmentation, but these processes often remain enigmatic and underspecified. What is being fragmented in the psyche? Are there stable results of the psychic fragmentation? How can we qualify them, especially when they do not map onto Freud's id, ego and superego? And what does it mean to work psychoanalytically with the fragments?

While I will hold these questions close throughout the book, I would like to take a moment to orient the reader to its matter. Let us focus on a detail of an ancient Roman mosaic, 'The Unswept Room' [*Asàrotos òikos*], reproduced below. In this extraordinary mosaic – dating from the time of Hadrian and (re-)found in 1833 between the gates of San Sebastiano and San Paolo in Rome, in a vineyard – a puzzle is put together from around twelve million small cubes of marble and of multicoloured molten glass, making up a composition of around four metres by four metres. With great detail and subtlety, the mosaic depicts remains, part-objects, fragments, leftovers. Leaning in, we discover snail shells and molluscs, a strawberry and some cherries, a chicken bone, apple peelings, seashells, the remains of a lobster, a lettuce leaf, a part of a lemon, fish bones and nutshells. All these unorderly objects and remains, sprinkled across the floor, seem to suggest an abundant feast that happened in another time. The figures of the mosaic each have their own shadow, making them stand out, and inviting anyone stepping across it to walk in between the part-objects scattered across the floor. This book is akin to walking across this mosaic: encountering at every step unusual or unknown or ambiguous fragments, arranged in a composition that does not seem obvious or orderly at first, and referencing complicated times and intricate scenes.

There is an important detail about orientation here: I put together for the reader something that resembles much more a *mosaic* or a *table* than a *tableau.* The *table* involves walking as a multi-sensorial and corporeal act, and also some form of engagement of the walker in the landscape that is being traversed. The *tableau*, by contrast, involves contemplation at a distance, or gazing at something that is situated in front of a viewer, who is thus external to the landscape being contemplated.

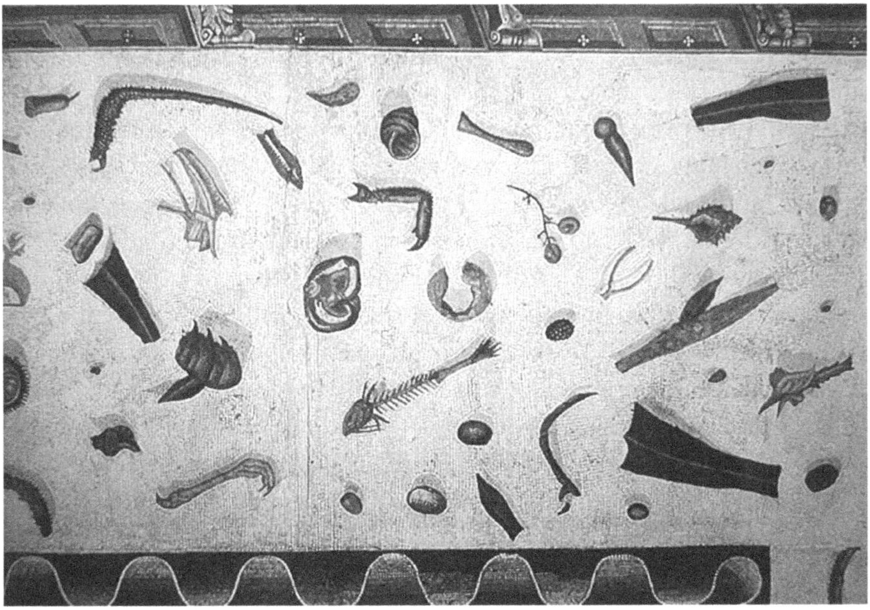

Figure 0.1 'The Unswept Room' Mosaic Detail (Vigna Lupi, Rome, Second Century CE), Musei Vaticani, Museo Gregoriano Profano, Rome.

Photograph by the Author.

Georges Didi-Huberman follows the implications of montage as an epistemological, ethical and artistic act, moving away from a single *tableau*, closed in upon itself and defined by its origin in the work of an author-genius, to the simpler and more disparate *table* or *plate* (Didi-Huberman, 2018, p. 8) which has no point of origin. As Didi-Huberman (2018, p. 47) writes:

> the prestigious French word *tableau* comes directly from an extremely banal Latin word, *tabula*, which simply means a plank or a board (*planche* in French). A board on which to do all kinds of things: to write, to count, to play, to eat, to arrange, to disarrange. [...] The tableau is a work, a result on which everything has always already been played out; the table is a device on which everything can always be played again. A tableau is hung in a museum; a table is reused constantly for new feasts, new configurations.

The plate or table (or, in our case, the mosaic representing the remains of a feast) also brings a renunciation of any visual unity or single temporal anchor: it is a space where several time threads cross and confront each other.

I would thus orient the reader to approach this book as if arranging objects on a table, or walking across a mosaic of remains, rather than standing in front of a picture, gazing at it and interpreting it. In a sense, this is an invitation to the reader to make their own montage of the fragments I am bringing, and, in the process of piecing them together, to experiment with producing a transformation of the experience of suffering by creating the possibility of (a partial) working-through and also by allowing the creation of new and surprising forms of life. The suffering I am referring to here is in itself defined as a transmission: it is the suffering belonging to patients; to the ones who came before them; to the clinicians who sit with them in the psychoanalytic consulting room; and to the space between the patients and the psychoanalysts.

In writing this book, I became more and more curious about montage as an artistic technique and I wondered what it means to create a *clinical* montage. Montage works by transforming the legibility and intelligibility of suffering, allowing the maker to shift their understanding of this suffering. The transformation occurs when moving between the different fragments that compose the montage, traversing the gaps that open up when we bring disparate things closer together. At the *threshold* between the different elements of the montage, vibrating with traces, marks, inscriptions, vestiges and memories, the montage-maker can see an event anew. It is the very intersection between past, present and future that invites a shift in perspectives. In the gap or on the threshold, one can better listen to the messages of the Other and to the singularity of their traces. I stress from the onset that the montage I speak of is a form of labour rather than one of exuberant play. The fragments resist, do not fit well together, or hold together in a composition that is unstable.

There are important ethical implications in deciding to pay attention to fragments and discarded psychic things. It instates *reusing* and *repurposing* as a core psychic practice. Drawing on insights from queer phenomenology (with Sara Ahmed), I often wonder in these pages about what is behind, beneath or below the table (rather than on the table, in front of us, in full display). To return to the mosaic I mentioned above, I wonder not only about what is in the mosaic, but also in the shadows of the part-objects of the mosaic. The psychoanalytic process can thus appear as a form of *gleaning*. As Laura Mulvey writes about gleaning, the practice 'gives a cultural lineage to the process of collecting, accumulating, sifting through and recycling discarded materials' (2017, p. 4). There is a feminist aspect to collecting the unwanted residue, the apparently trivial things, the scraps, the 'outcast' objects. For me, this is a necessary exploration for *another* psychoanalysis, a *minor psychoanalysis,* which is capable of considering marginal lives, non-normative sexualities, and generally psychic life beyond the phallus.

This minor psychoanalysis is in itself rendered plural: there is not one single revision that I propose, but several figurations making up a minor composition. There is a *psychoanalysis of scars*, held together by a vocabulary of wounds, lesions and scar-tissues. Here, the attention goes to the scar-tissue resulting from the encounter with the Other, out of which both memory and the ego are made. There is a *psychoanalysis of organs*, animated by an interest in radical plasticity, in the surprising modes of psychic splitting that result from the scene of trauma, and in 'semifluid' bodies and organs that reshape, retract, and grow new parts. Here, the guiding question is 'what can an organ *do*?' or 'what can a fragment *do*?' There is an *eventful psychoanalysis*, which acknowledges contingency and the possibility of radical transformation, and which is interested in catastrophes and the ways in which trauma can be both destructive and creative. Finally, there is a *blue psychoanalysis*, proposing an unusual perspectival move: starting from the sea, from moving waters and from sea critters. Listening closely to sea critters means learning from their breathing techniques, their modes of memory, and their ways of splitting themselves into fragments. Considered together, these four modalities are a prism for a minor composition.

In assembling this minor psychoanalysis, I am in constant dialogue with psychoanalyst Sándor Ferenczi, in both matters of theory and clinical insights. Ferenczi is a thinker of the Budapest School of Psychoanalysis, a contemporary of Freud, and an 'outcast' himself, for several decades, after his break from Freud.[1] This volume is written in between two consulting rooms – Ferenczi's and my own – perhaps sharing a waiting room across time.

The pages opening before you, reader, are an exercise in the clinical imagination on trauma, radical plasticity and psychic fragmentation. Over the years, I closely followed Sándor Ferenczi's revisions to the work of

Sigmund Freud. I see these revisions as a *metapsychology of fragmented psyches*. For Ferenczi, psychic fragmentation is a ubiquitous operation of the psyche. What happens if we lean into the fragments, if we let ourselves be surprised by the multiplicity of forms of fragmentation, and if we qualify and describe the fragments and their lives? What if we follow Ferenczi along his vocabulary on fractures, splits, atomisations, pulverisations, leakages, detritus, shattering of psychic matter into particles without form, but also new formations, protective membranes, expansions, contagions, and inner growths? To the Freudian vocabulary of splitting [*spaltung*] Ferenczi thus adds a new register of terms, which I discuss as processes of psychic de-materialisation, but also as processes of psychic reconstruction. Considering novel psychic processes such as atomisation and pulverisation is an important step in working psychoanalytically with radically fragmented psychic states.

The theory of trauma is analogous to a theory of montage. The Ferenczian subject bears certain structural similarities to a montage made out of cut-out fragments. For Ferenczi, the organism itself is thought of as prepared for art: ready for recombinations, permutations, complex analogies, imports and implantations. Surprising modes of psychic splitting result from the scene of trauma. With the traumatic attack, bodies and organs become 'semifluid' and change their shape or grow new curious parts. Ferenczi (1932, p. 7) calls post-traumatic fragments and organs 'semisubstances', in the sense that they 'have the extraordinary or wonderfully pleasing quality of being both body and mind simultaneously, that is, of expressing wishes, sensations of pleasure-unpleasure, or even complicated thoughts, through changes in their structure or function'. Fragments have lives of their own: they 'speak' in a different voice and in the consulting room these different voices can become discernible.

In thinking through trauma, I start with the question: 'What does it mean to have survived a psychic catastrophe?' The catastrophe is not a singular, unitary event, but a *scene* where qualitative forces hold together. The fragments resulting from the catastrophe make an arrangement, a composition, a relational ensemble. Or, a montage. Trauma is not an irrevocably broken symbol or the collapse of all capacity for symbolisation. Trauma is perhaps an interrupted symbol, bearing the mark of an intrusion by the other. But after this interruption, or syncope, what comes is a reorganisation *of* the fragments and a reconstruction *from* the fragments – sometimes even an extraordinary acceleration of recombinatory capacities; or 'hyper-faculties', as Ferenczi would call them. Something dies, but something else is re-enlivened, vivified, accelerated.

One point of return in the book is the position of the psychoanalyst. I experiment with theorising a non-Oedipal position of the analyst, one that is not stuck in the mummy–daddy–child triangle. Indeed, Ferenczi's constructions on psychoanalytic technique offer a rich starting point, thinking through the possibility of mutuality in the psychoanalytic dyad, the invisible power structure of the psychoanalytic dispositif, the elasticity of psychoanalytic technique, the plasticity of the position of the analyst, and the therapeutic value of phenomena of regression in the psychoanalytic frame. Building on this, I work towards a *substance-centred view of the analyst's position* that transcends the need to be coded as parental or familial roles. In his 1968 book *The Basic Fault*, psychoanalyst Michael Balint, a close collaborator of Ferenczi, voices this surprising post-humanist and substance-sensitive view:

> The air is not an object but a substance, like water or milk. [...] there are a few – not many – more such substances, among them the elements of the pre-Socratic philosophers: water, earth, and fire; with some others used in present-day guidance clinics, such as sand and water or plasticine. The chief characteristic is their indestructibility. You can build a castle out of wet sand, then destroy it, and the sand will still be there; you can stop the jet of water coming from a tap but, as soon as you take your finger away, the jet is there again, and so on'.
>
> (Bálint, 1968, p. 136)

Balint goes on to argue in favour of assimilating the position of the analyst to such primary substances. The analyst must be extraordinarily plastic or pliable; they must also show endurance, or even, as Balint shows, display a special kind of substance-indestructibility: one that sustains what is being built, without showing invulnerability or superiority. To return to my response to my patient Ava's question above – 'Do you know that painting by Dali? It's a Renaissance girl-head exploding?' – I note that one of my first associations was with an image of the wheelbarrow contained in the painting, and not with any maternal or paternal role in the transference. In this instance, the question 'What can a wheelbarrow do?' is much more energising and significant than the question 'Am I a maternal or a paternal analyst?'

Before stepping into the chapters, I would like to tie some methodological threads. My first note on method is about the practice of *rereading*. In the past thirteen years, an important part of my thinking and writing has had to do with constantly rereading the work of Sándor Ferenczi. For around fifty years, between his premature death in 1933 and up to the 1980s, Ferenczi was an impossible 'object' in psychoanalysis, a traumatically forgotten thinker, after a break from Freud. It was thus necessary to relearn to read and reread Ferenczi. I now understand this rereading as a form of intensification. The ethos, the orientation behind the rereading I offer is that the insight being assembled is not only to be 'used' but *played*, perhaps like a musical instrument, and passed on, passed forward. I reread Ferenczi every year not to contribute to Ferenczi's legacy, but precisely in order to uproot him, to allow all the strangeness, and the untamed, and the unacademic parts to emerge from the text. I reread Ferenczi, so as to relink different sections in a new way each time, making visible new relations that are often disturbing. By rereading Ferenczi, I reread the twentieth century afresh, and Central and Eastern Europe, and the traumas of the great wars and their military, social, political and aesthetic ruin. To reread thus does not mean making everything return to its place, but precisely intensifying what is ossified, or deadened, or still. A rereading of this sort means descending into dark times, facing the spectralities of the text, and not only its clarities or illuminations.

This rereading in itself functions as a montage. It involves wondering not only what Ferenczi *thought*, but also what he had in front of him on his worktable. I have often asked myself what this table might have contained. We have fewer historical records than in the case of Freud to reconstitute this surface, since Ferenczi's house on the Sunny Hill in Budapest was bombed and looted during WWII. There is thus more space for the imagination and also a necessity to go through debris. I trust Ferenczi's table contained several non-psychoanalytic objects and writings, perhaps books in popular biology[2] and poetry books. I imagine on his table we would have found an as-yet-unpublished manuscript by Sándor Márai and a musical score by Béla Bartók.

My rereading of Ferenczi was possible in the thirteen years that came before 2025 also because of several other rereadings that preceded it. As

I write, we've known many waves of a Ferenczi revival, from appreciating his contribution to metapsychology and trauma theory;[3] to theorising the drives and problematising the dualism of the drives;[4] to renewing our vocabulary on psychoanalytic technique (where ideas such as 'tact' and 'mutuality' are crucial) and on the importance of countertransference of the analyst to their analysand;[5] to reconfiguring the relationship between psyche and soma as well as between psychoanalysis, medicine, and biology;[6] to reconsidering the Oedipus complex and insisting on the importance of early object relations and regressive states;[7] to opening the possibility of new 'Ferenczian' questions in social theory, in cultural theory and in critical theory.[8] Within this rich revival, a few voices are present in this book even when they are not cited: Antal Bókay, Jay Frankel, Giselle Galdi, Adrienne Harris, Galina Hristeva, Endre Koritar and Judit Szekacs.

My second note on method is about the practice of *co-montage*. As I mentioned already, the rereading I am talking about is of the labouring kind, involving an encounter with spectralities and the dark side of texts. To traverse this darkness, a kind of solidarity in rereading is needed: a co-production, a co-affectation, a coalition, something more marked than just co-authorship. A co-montage. The co-montage I would like to invoke here is the one I created with Jenny Willner and Jakob Staberg through the book we published in 2023, *Ferenczi Dialogues: On Trauma and Catastrophe* (Soreanu et al., 2023). Our book was the result of a three-year-long dialogue about the philosophical, political and clinical implications of ideas and images of catastrophe in Ferenczi's work, which grew from our different disciplinary points of view and against the background of social history. We read Ferenczi in an interdisciplinary landscape – including social sciences, literary theory, psychoanalytic theory, and clinical practice. *Ferenczi Dialogues* was planned and written during the COVID-19 pandemic, finished during the months in which war in Europe became a dominating subject again. For the three of us, this book was a form of surviving by making a montage, assembling something from fragments, corresponding between different countries and disciplinary contexts, meeting on the screen. Each of our individual rereadings of Ferenczi changed when encountering the rereadings of the others. I don't think we wrote *Ferenczi Dialogues* as Ferenczi's children, but as more ambiguous kin across time. What connected us is an interest in radical plasticity or the propensity of the mind to undergo change. This interest lingers on. After co-authoring

Ferenczi Dialogues, I am in a constant co-montage with Jenny Willner and Jakob Staberg, as their own writings un-do and re-do my own. They are both active principles in the book you are holding in your hands.

My third – and perhaps most important – note on method has to do with the place of patients in creating any sort of psychoanalytic knowledge. Psychoanalyst Arnold W. Rachman, in his book *Elizabeth Severn: The 'Evil Genius' of Psychoanalysis*, traces the encounter between Ferenczi and one of his key patients, also the protagonist of Ferenczi's *Clinical Diary*, Elizabeth Severn. In Rachman's account, Ferenczi and his patient Severn appear as a creative dyad. What we usually regard as Ferenczi's 'trauma theory' is treated as a co-creation as well. Without Severn's experimentations with self-hypnotic trance states, Ferenczi would perhaps not have grasped the importance of regression and reliving in the psychoanalytic frame or the importance of the analysis of countertransference.

There is another question that opens here. My writing, as a psychoanalyst, is *full* of my patients, and I am yet to invent forms of thinking and writing to appropriately traverse this particular kind of fullness. The clinical writing that you will encounter in this book, reader, happens in a near-impossible fold. On the one hand, it is hard to imagine any psychoanalytic transmission without clinical cases and vignettes. On the other hand, while writing clinical vignettes, it is of stringent importance to consider the ethics of clinical writing. I don't mean this in the narrow sense of respecting anonymity, asking for consent, or writing composite or semi-fictionalised cases – which are of course crucial ethical acts in themselves. I mean that while clinical *insight* is predicated on a co-montage of the psychoanalytic dyad, clinical *writing* is often structurally predicated on reducing something that was co-produced to being inscribed by one single voice: the voice of the analyst. In other words, there is a displacement at play in clinical writing. There is no easy way to address this impasse, which is why the clinical writing in this book is deliberately hybrid and pluri-genre. I not only resort to composite and fictionalised cases, but, in some instances, the vignettes break down into poetry-in-prose (see the first vignette in Chapter 1), so as to mark this nearly impossible kind of inscription. Here, reader, as you will see, paragraphs dissolve, and rhythms matter. In other instances (see Chapter 3), I make an imaginary alliance with fiction writer Amélie Nothomb. In her novels, I found a kind of internal ear, listening to the various voices of psychic fragmentation. The fragments speak, suffer, or are in dialogue with one another. It is as if we were able to hear the psychic scenes and discern the elements that make up these scenes. Entering a 'transcript' of psychic fragments, we get to hear entire parts of the psyche growing up too fast, or lagging behind, or stepping outside time, or attacking other times of the psyche, or eternalising the present, or reliving a moment of the traumatic past. This is another tactic to address the impasses of clinical writing.

The matter of this book has been clarified through clinical-theoretical teaching, over a decade, in several countries and contexts: from psychoanalytic societies to universities and cultural institutions. The hidden subtitle of the book could be 'The Ferenczi Lectures', capturing not one single series of lectures but several, intersecting and overlayered. I owe many insights to my students and their questions, which pulled new threads of thought and opened new associations. As Inayatullah observes, 'if teaching is possible at all, it occurs from body to body' (2013, p. 153). This is even more the case for clinical teaching. While I teach, I move and walk quite a lot, so my body performs, misperforms, reperforms, or searches, as I transmit Ferenczi's trauma theory and my understanding of the psychic life of fragments. While I teach, I also draw a lot on the blackboard, looking for more condensed ways to represent an often-intricate idea or grammar, such as the psychic positions of the scene of trauma. The schemas of Chapter 1 of the book took shape during teaching, in a way that involves my own body and the bodies of those who were listening and engaging.

As the subtitle announces, this book is also about the experience of time in psychoanalysis. It is an experiment in phenomenology, tracing different qualities of time, as they present themselves in the consulting room, in the space between the couch and the psychoanalytic chair. There are resonances here with the work of phenomenological psychiatry, especially Eugène Minkowski's (1933) *Lived Time: Phenomenological and Psychopathological Studies*. The psychic life of fragments has a temporal dimension, and in what follows I trace the times of fragments. As Gilles Deleuze (1988) stated, time is 'a polyphony of polyphonies': it contains an infinity of worlds. In these pages, psychoanalysis becomes a machine for further differentiating, qualifying and describing psychic times. This starts with Freud and with the innovative temporality of *Nachträglichkeit*, or afterwardsness, or après-coup. It can continue with Ferenczi, who orients us to the 'wild' temporalities of psychic fragments. To be fragmented means to function across several temporal threads, which often interact in a violent manner, by attacking or dislocating one another.

Time is no neutral matter. It is an issue of power and normativity. Normative temporal regimes are not only patriarchal in nature, but also racialised, heteronormative, and cisnormative, and they function to oppress and exclude subjects who do not conform to the conventions of Western modernity on time, progress and development. A linear temporal regime lies at the heart of modern conceptions and practices of time, where 'uncivilised' others are figured as stuck in the past, in the cyclical time of nature or of mythology. As Walter Mignolo (2011) shows, the mainstream modern time as experienced today 'is a result and a consequence of the colonial matrix of power'. According to this logic, Europe lives in the present, while the rest of the world lives in the past. Aníbal Quijano (2009) argues that modernity is built on a linear, one-directional evolutionism from some state of nature to modern European society, which also distortedly relocates cultural differences by temporally displacing non-Europeans into the past. Thinking with Elizabeth Freeman (2010), we can bring into focus the vocabularies that pertain to this normative temporal regime, which she names 'chrononormativity'. This refers to institutional forces coming to operate like 'somatic facts' and to 'forms of temporal experience that seem natural to those whom they privilege' (2010, p. 3). It is important to note that as a modern discourse, psychoanalysis cannot fully transcend chrononormativity, and the opposition between the primitive and the civilised has been one of the points of legitimate critique to Freud.

But psychoanalysis also enables and works with temporalities that escape chrononormativity. Katie Gentile (2024) talks about 'dense temporalities', tracing the interwoven nature of times (past, present and future), beyond linear progression. She envisions dense temporalities as 'the perpetual motions of time and space vertically through past, present and future generations of all beings and matter, as well as horizontally, encapsulating all bodies, objects, environments, etc. and their various rhythms of temporality' (2024, p. 177). This allows for imagining agency as more-than-human, and also complex 'transferences' between generations of kin, which share intimate knowledge and relatedness. Lisa Baraitser (2017) writes about suspended time, or time that is not flowing and appears to have become stuck. She asks how we 'take care' of time and gestures to the realm of an obdurate time that refuses to pass: waiting, delaying, staying, remaining, enduring, returning and repeating. Psychoanalysis itself is such a practice of 'taking care' of time, while also living with slow time, or with time that appears to be 'wasted'.

What brings these perspectives together is non-linear thinking, but also a queer-phenomenological sensibility to what is *behind, beneath* or *below* the 'table', rather than in full display. Thinking about queer temporalities, Fanny Söderbäck (2019, p. 19) reminds us that they 'swerve and interrupt, stretch and bend, wrinkle and fold, halt and diverge, redeploy and twist, are "out of joint" and uncanny while attending to gaps, failures, and slippages in the seemingly smooth texture of heterolinear time'. While psychoanalysis holds some important resources for 'queering' time, it has not always, in theory and in practice, followed through with this potentiality. Indeed, as thinkers such as Judith Butler, Patricia Gherovici, Avgi Saketopoulou, Ann Pellegrini and Paul B. Preciado[9] remind us, many psychoanalysts – and psychoanalysis as an institution – are failing trans and queer lives. Discourses of 'arrested development' or 'just a phase' are projected onto gay, lesbian, trans and other subjects that are associated with non-normative genders, identities and experiences. These projections are a source of much harm and injury. They are also flattening and re-folding psychoanalysis into the seemingly smooth texture of heterolinear time that hides away all its racialised and patriarchal violence.

In the face of this, moments of queering psychoanalysis are precious (see Giffney & Watson, 2017). They reinstate the plurality and internal differentiation of time, or, following Deleuze (1988), they reinstate time as 'a polyphony of polyphonies'. My contemporary dialogue with Sándor Ferenczi pays attention to small moments of obliqueness, transversality, interruption, and also to stretching and bending, wrinkling and folding, redeploying and twisting, diverging and disrupting, failing and slipping, reusing and repurposing, or just going through debris. I don't aim to suggest that psychoanalysis has always been queer, or that Ferenczi was a queer thinker, but rather that he can be an 'accomplice' for queer thinking and for a minor psychoanalysis-to-come.

This book does not contain an extensive biographical account of Ferenczi: instead, I propose to register some of his own orientations to queer objects, in minor traces. Let us turn to a very early text by Ferenczi, which is a kind of inter-form: part object of dialogue with the medical establishment of his times, part theoretical intervention, part activist piece taking a stance in the defence of homosexuals. In 1906, in Budapest, the year after Freud wrote his first version of the 'Three Essays…', Sándor Ferenczi (1906) presents the text 'Intermediary Sexual States' ['Szexuális átmeneti fokozatokról'] before the Medical Association of Budapest. At this time Ferenczi defines himself as a neurologist, and he has not yet met Freud. We do not yet have an English translation of this extraordinary text; we only have Hungarian and French versions. It is worth noting that in 1905 Ferenczi became the Budapest representative of the International Humanitarian Committee for the Defence of Homosexuals, created by the prominent Berlin sexologist Magnus Hirschfeld. He signed petitions calling for legal reforms around the criminalisation of homosexuality and he published the talk we are looking at here. Freud expressed his sympathy for this Committee, but he did not wish to be associated with the initiatives for legal reform.

In 1906, Ferenczi speaks to the medical establishment in the hope that it would tolerate an intervention, an incision, a political breach, an activist statement in defence of a marginalised and oppressed group. As Ferenczi writes:

> According to Hirschfeld, himself backed up by eminent physicians, individuals do not all progress toward a determined masculine or feminine type. There exist in certain cases certain intermediary forms between the two sexes. In the psycho-physiological organisation of such individuals, the masculine and feminine traits are intermixed.
>
> (Ferenczi, 1906, p. 244, my translation from the French edition)

The theoretical intervention in this short piece has a queer orientation: Ferenczi seems to speak from a place beyond the phallus. In the text, he differentiates between *primary sexual traits* (genitals, which he analyses as fundamentally hermaphroditic in nature since the first days of embryonic life); *secondary sexual traits* (gained by bodies in puberty, but occurring in surprising mixes); and, remarkably, *tertiary sexual traits*, or *the psychological character*. This tertiary category involves, on the one hand, the subjective, lived, phantasised experiencing of both primary sexual traits and secondary sexual traits (or, we might say, *'lived' gender*); and sexual attraction, love (or, we might say, with Freud, *object choice*). Although he does place a male and a female character as two types of this tertiary layer, again, remarkably, a study of many cases shows us an extreme *variety* of intermediary states, more or less feminine men and more or less masculine women, where the individual's sexual being results from a *modulation* of primary, secondary and tertiary sexual traits. What Ferenczi writes is an anticipation of Patricia Gherovici's (2017b) succinct formulation on sexual difference: sex needs to be symbolised, while gender needs to be embodied.

In support of his thesis on tertiary sexual traits, Ferenczi also brings a letter written by a transvestite, who describes the (voluptuous but also ordinary) experience of wearing women's clothes, also making a case that the transvestite's seduction of their object of love is in effect, and if seen from close up, no different from the seduction of a man by a woman. There is nothing outrageous about it. I think Ferenczi's commentary on this letter is a moment of queer spectrality (Dinshaw et al., 2007, p. 178): a moment when the affective force of the past erupts into the present, speaking of a desire from another time and placing a demand on the present in the form of an ethical imperative. How to write a new theory of sexuality beyond the phallus? How to dismantle all-powerful fathers, patriarchal and transphobic orientations, including in the work of our dreams? It is on the basis of minor moments, such as his orientation in this 1906 text, that Ferenczi can be part of a composition beyond heterolinear time.

*

In Chapter 1 of the book, I create a montage that takes the reader into the atmosphere of living among fragments, scraps, detritus – but also new growths, protective membranes and contagions. I also propose a reconstruction of Ferenczi's trauma theory, following his insights on psychic fragmentation, and I revisit the grammar of the scene of trauma. This results in a metapsychology of fragmented psyches. In the first section, I ask what it means to practice a *psychoanalysis of scars*, paying attention to wounds, lesions and scar-tissues. I read trauma not as a dead space and the end of symbolisation, but as the precipitation of representation, images, capacities of relating, specific faculties and even hyper-faculties. I follow Ferenczi's insight that memory operates both through the id and through the ego, producing two distinct modalities of making inscriptions, or two registers of memory: the memory of the id and the memory of the ego. This new 'situation of memory' intervenes in how we think of representation, language, symbol and symptom. I explore Ferenczi's little-known vocabulary of pleasure (including the 'pleasure of resemblance', the 'pleasure in repetition', and the 'pleasure in rediscovery'), which contributes to composing a non-dualistic picture of the drives. To Ferenczi's vocabulary of pleasure I add the *pleasure of analogy*, which is a doubly relational pleasure: the pleasure of establishing a relation between two relations. Through a clinical vignette, I explore the nature of symbolisation and the way an analyst's missing word is implicated in making sense of a symptom.

In the second section of the chapter, I ask: what does it mean that psychic fragments have a life? To address the phenomenological gap in psychoanalysis around psychic splitting, I unpack Ferenczi's unique vocabulary of fragmentation. Staging a dialogue between Melanie Klein and Sándor Ferenczi, I propose the distinction between 'mundane splitting' (or splitting *by* the ego) and 'eventful splitting' (or splitting *of* the ego). Furthermore, I explore two other facets of a minor psychoanalysis: *blue psychoanalysis* and a *psychoanalysis of organs*.

In the third section, I enter the domain of an *eventful psychoanalysis* and revise the scene of trauma, following oblique lines and uncommon transversal trajectories. I offer my reading of the psychic grammar of the confusion of tongues as an asymmetric encounter between two psychic registers. Ferenczi's trauma theory is also a theory of the subject, and it opens up the exploration of new psychic processes, such as traumatic imitation and the identification with the aggressor – but also ex-corporation and resistance to the identification with the aggressor. I show that, for Ferenczi, the child is not simply looking in on a scene in which the adults are acting, but she is included in the trauma scene. Revisiting the scene of trauma has implications for how we conceive of the position of the analyst: this position is oblique, as the analyst is *never only within* the scene of trauma, identified with one or the other of its positions, and *never only outside* the scene of trauma, looking in from above as a distant observer.

*

Chapter 2 of the book engages Ferenczi's revision to the Freudian construction of the death drive and life drive. I follow Ferenczi's innovative orientations in relation to the drives and their ramifications for psychoanalytic theory and practice today. I ask what we lose with Freud's (1920) event-text 'Beyond the Pleasure Principle' and what can still be imagined in the horizon of the drives. Firstly, Freud does not construct theoretical 'inheritors' for what, until 1920, he referred to as 'the ego instincts'. Secondly, there is a strong link in Freudian thinking between the compulsion to repeat and the death drive. By reading Ferenczi's metapsychological insights, I aim to pluralise our thinking on repetition and ask what a Ferenczian *Nachträglichkeit* might look like. I discuss a new psychic time, *the time of reliving*. Through this idea, we can give a different meaning to the Freudian series repetition/remembering/reliving. I trace the genealogy of the time of reliving in relation to the scene of trauma and I connect it to the event of survival. In a clinical vignette, I look at the way the time of reliving operates in the consulting room in moments that Ferenczi calls 'neo-catharsis'.

Finally, I explore Ferenczi's ideas on 'the feminine principle', showing how it intervenes in the sphere of the drives. Ferenczi articulates a vocabulary in which terms such as conciliation, endurance of suffering, selflessness, appeasement, adaptation, renunciation, self-denial, and compromise, percolate and are arranged in a surprising way with a direct relation to Ferenczi's trauma theory. The feminine principle brings a rethinking of the reality principle, a re-evaluation of the duality of the drives and of the unexplored forms of the life drive. In *The Clinical Diary,* Ferenczi presents us with a particular modification to the sphere of the death drive/life drive dualism: he renames them the 'drive of self-assertion' and the 'drive of conciliation'. The 'selflessness' he evokes includes the 'selflessness' of organs: it describes a psychic state that considers otherness and the relationship to the environment. The 'drive for conciliation' expresses the fact that, in order to survive as any sort of individuality, one needs to practice a kind of politics of self-limitation. These ideas on 'the feminine principle' are tied in with a revision of the theory of sexuality. Ferenczi invites us to democratise forms of erotism: he has in mind a clever combination of mechanisms of pleasure and rich mixtures or transpositions of the erotic in psychic life.

*

In Chapter 3, we meet 'Orpha' and Orphic temporalities. Orpha is a new psychic agency that takes shape in Ferenczi's late work, especially in the *Clinical Diary*, constituting an important revision to Freudian metapsychology. Orpha is a psychic system not just a mechanism of defence. Under the strength of the traumatic attack, the psyche is forced to devise new ways to care for itself, and at times the only way to do so is by fragmenting itself into *parts that care* and *parts to be cared for*. We are in the terrain of a tragic narcissism of fragments, where the self does not take itself for an object, like in the Freudian story of narcissism, but the self treats one of its parts as an 'other' and takes *it* as an object. A new optics to the scene of trauma is created through the split between a part of the self that is undergoing the aggression or being overwhelmed and a part of the self that is watching all this from above. I show how Ferenczi arrived at his formulation of 'Orpha' as a co-creation with his patient Elizabeth Severn. I examine Ferenczi's 'pre-Orphic' vocabulary, centred on ideas such as 'getting beside oneself', 'traumatic progression', 'autotomy', 'neo-formations', 'teleplastia', the 'wise baby', and 'reconstruction'. Drawing on clinical vignettes and literary fragments, I conjure Orphic psychic atmospheres populated by guardian angels, improbable forms of survival, protective bladders, tubes and severed organs. I also discuss the psychic temporalities of Orpha and ask: how are Orphic times experienced in the psyche and how do they appear in the transference, in the consulting room? I reference a particular kind of 'eternal present' as the main temporality of Orpha. In this eternal present, the subject seemingly iterates: 'I can do everything' or 'I can do anything'.

*

Chapter 4 of the book is dedicated to tracing the psychoanalyst's times or the 'metapsychology of the analyst's mental process during analysis' (Ferenczi, 1928, p. 98). Ideas of time in the psychoanalytic process function as *meta-constructions*: they organise the scene. Meta-constructions are the grids within which analysts place other constructions during the analytic session. Countering the insistence on the atemporal nature of the drive and on the 'timelessness of the unconscious', I qualify the different threads of time that organise the psychoanalytic encounter. I show that Ferenczi has a unique approach to time, opening up to the mythological, historical, and intersubjective dimensions of time. I discuss three threads of time: a tangent (or originary time), a segment (or organic time), and a meandering line (or pulsating time). I bring a clinical vignette to capture these different qualities of time in the consulting room. I then follow the implications of this plurality of times for the position of the analyst, drawing on Ferenczi's vocabulary on technique, which includes mutuality, elasticity and horizontality. The analyst's intervention is that of inhabiting, with the patient, a polyphonic temporality, one where there is the present, but also the deep past, and recent past, and conditional future, and distant future, and many other times that are yet to be named.

Notes

1 See Staberg (2023a).
2 See Willner (2023).
3 See Bokanowski (2004), Bókay (2015), Bonomi (2003), Borgogno (2007), Dupont (2010), Frankel (1998), Haynal (2014) and Soreanu (2018a).
4 See Avello (1998), Cabré (2009), Dal Molin et al. (2023), Soreanu (2017), Staberg (2023b) and Staberg (2024).
5 See Falzeder (2010), Haynal (1999), Hirsch (2018) and Koritar (2022).
6 See Hristeva (2013) and Willner (2023). A double special issue of the journal RISS was dedicated to Ferenczi's take on biology: *RISS. Zeitschrift für Psychoanalyse: Bioanalysen I* 94, 2021, and *Bioanalysen II* 95, 2022.
7 See Stewart (2012).
8 See Salgó (2014), Gandesha (2018), Erős (2018), Soreanu (2018b) and Kupermann (2022).
9 See Butler (2024), Gherovici (2017a), Saketopoulou & Pellegrini (2023) and Preciado (2021).

References

Avello, J. J. (1998). Metapsychology in Ferenczi: Death instinct or death passion? *International Forum of Psychoanalysis*, 7: 229–234.

Bálint, M. (1968). *The Basic Fault. Therapeutic Aspects of Regression*. London: Tavistock.

Baraitser, L. (2017). *Enduring Time*. London: Bloomsbury.

Bokanowski, T. (2004). Splitting, fragmenting, and mental agony: The clinical thinking of Sándor Ferenczi. *International Forum of Psychoanalysis*, 13(1–2): 20–25.

Bókay, A. (2015). The child as a traumatic self-component in Ferenczi's later psychoanalysis. *American Journal of Psychoanalysis*, 75(1): 46–56.

Bonomi, C. (2003). Between symbol and antisymbol: The meaning of trauma reconsidered. *International Forum of Psychoanalysis*, 12(1): 17–21.

Borgogno, F. (2007). Ferenczi's clinical and theoretical conception of trauma: A brief introductory map. *American Journal of Psychoanalysis*, 67: 141–149.

Butler, J. (2024). *Who's Afraid of Gender?* London: Penguin Books.

Cabré, L. J. M. (2009). Ferenczi's 'Feminine principle': A feminine version of the death drive. *American Imago*, 66(4): 411–418.

Dal Molin, E. C., Coelho Junior, N. E., & Cromberg, R. U. (2023). Ferenczi's variations on the death drive. *American Journal of Psychoanalysis*, 83(2): 231–249.

Deleuze, G. (1988). *Le Pli: Leibniz et la Baroque*. Paris: Minuit.

Didi-Huberman, G. (2018). *Atlas, Or the Anxious Gay Science*. Chicago, IL: University of Chicago Press.

Dinshaw, C., Edelman, L., Ferguson, R. A., Freccero, C., Freeman, E., Halberstam, J., Jagose, A., Nealon, C., & Nguyen, T. H. (2007). Theorizing queer temporalities: A roundtable discussion. *GLQ: A Journal of Lesbian and Gay Studies*, 13(2): 177–195.

Dupont, J. (2010). The concept of trauma according to Ferenczi and its effects on subsequent psychoanalytic research. *International Forum of Psychoanalysis*, 7(4): 235–241.

Erős, F. (2018). Against violence: Ferenczi and liberal socialism. In: A. Dimitrijević, G. Cassullo, & J. Frankel (eds), *Ferenczi's Influence on Contemporary Psychoanalytic Traditions* (pp. 248–254). London: Routledge.

Falzeder, E. (2010). Sándor Ferenczi between orthodoxy and heterodoxy. *American Imago*, 66(4): 395–404.

Ferenczi, S. (1906). États sexuels intermédiaires [Intermediary Sexual States]. In: *Les écrits de Budapest [The Budapest Writings]* (pp. 243–255). Paris: EPEL, 1994.

Ferenczi, S. (1928). The elasticity of psycho-analytic technique. In: *Final contributions to the Problems and Methods of Psycho-analysis* (transl. by E. Mosbacher, pp. 87–101). London: Karnac, 1994.

Ferenczi, S. (1932). *The Clinical Diary of Sándor Ferenczi*, ed. by J. Dupont (transl. by M. Bálint & N. Z. Jackson). Cambridge, MA: Harvard University Press, 1995.

Frankel, J. (1998). Ferenczi's trauma theory. *American Journal of Psychoanalysis*, 58(1): 41–61.

Freeman, E. (2010). *Time Binds: Queer Temporalities, Queer Histories*. Durham, NC: Duke University Press.

Freud, S. (1920). Beyond the pleasure principle. In: *Standard Edition* (Vol. 18, pp. 3–64). London: Hogarth Press.

Gandesha, S. (2018). Identifying with the aggressor. From the authoritarian to the neoliberal personality. *Constellations*, 25(1): 1–18.

Gentile, K. (2024). Destroying the 'human' for the survival of the world: A proposal for a temporally dense psychoanalytic subject. *Psychoanalytic Dialogues*, 34(2): 173–189.

Gherovici, P. (2017a). *Transgender Psychoanalysis: A Lacanian Perspective on Sexual Difference*. London & New York, NY: Taylor & Francis.

Gherovici, P. (2017b). Botched bodies: Inventing gender and constructing sex. In: V. Tsolas & C. Anzieu-Premmereur (eds), *A Psychoanalytic Exploration of the Body in Today's World* (pp. 159–173). London & New York, NY: Routledge.

Giffney, N., & Watson, E. (2017). *Clinical Encounters in Sexuality: Psychoanalytic Practice and Queer Theory*. New York, NY: Punctum Books.

Haynal, A. (1999). Countertransference in the work of Ferenczi. *American Journal of Psychoanalysis*, 59: 315–331.

Haynal, A. (2014). Trauma – revisited: Ferenczi and modern psychoanalysis. *Psychoanalytic Inquiry*, 34(2): 98–111.

Hirsch, I. (2018). Countertransference and the person of the therapist. In: A. Dimitrijević, G. Cassullo, & J. Frankel (eds), *Ferenczi's Influence on Contemporary Psychoanalytic Traditions* (pp. 165–168). London: Routledge.

Hristeva, G. (2013). 'Uterus loquitur': Trauma and the human organism in Ferenczi's 'physiology of pleasure'. *American Journal of Psychoanalysis*, 73(4): 339–352.

Inayatullah, N. (2013). Impossibilities: Generative misperformance and the movements of the teaching body. In: J. Edkins & A. Kear (eds), *International Politics and Performance: Critical Aesthetics and Creative Practice* (pp. 150–157). London: Routledge.

Koritar, E. (2022). Ferenczi's researches in technique. *American Journal of Psychoanalysis*, 82: 210–221.

Kupermann, D. (2022). Social trauma and testimony: A reading of Maryan S. Maryan's Notebooks inspired by Sándor Ferenczi. *American Journal of Psychoanalysis*, 82(2): 268–280.

Mignolo, W. D. (2011). *The Darker Side of Western Modernity: Global Futures, Decolonial Options*. Durham, NC: Duke University Press.

Minkowski, E. (1933). *Lived Time: Phenomenological and Psychological Studies* (transl. by N. Metzel). Evanston, IL: Northwestern University Press, 1970.

Mulvey, L. (2017). *Time at a Crossroads: Some Background Thoughts on Death 24 Times a Second: Stillness and the Moving Image in Relation to the Temporal Imaginaries of the Compilation Film*. Dora Volume One. Paper 6. https://www.dorichhousemuseum.org.uk/research-archive/dora-volume-one/

Preciado, P. B. (2021). *Can the Monster Speak? Report to an Academy of Psychoanalysts*. Pasadena, CA: Semiotext(e), Intervention Series No. 32.

Quijano, A. (2009). Coloniality of power, Eurocentrism, and Latin America. *Nepantia: Views from South*, 1(3): 533–580.

Saketopoulou, A., & Pellegrini, A. (2023). *Gender without Identity*. New York, NY: The Unconscious in Translation.

Salgó, E. (2014). *Psychoanalytic Reflections on Politics: Fatherlands in Mothers' Hands*. London & New York, NY: Routledge.

Söderbäck, F. (2019). *Revolutionary Time: On Time and Difference in Kristeva and Irigaray*. Albany, NY: State University of New York Press.

Soreanu, R., (2017). Something was lost in Freud's Beyond the pleasure principle: A Ferenczian reading. *American Journal of Psychoanalysis*, 77(3): 223–238.

Soreanu, R., (2018a). The psychic life of fragments: Splitting from Ferenczi to Klein. *American Journal of Psychoanalysis*, 78(4): 421–444.

Soreanu, R. (2018b). *Working-Through Collective Wounds: Trauma, Denial, Recognition in the Brazilian Uprising*. London: Palgrave Macmillan.

Soreanu, R., Staberg, J., & Willner, J. (2023). *Ferenczi Dialogues: On Trauma and Catastrophe*. Leuven: Leuven University Press.

Staberg, J. (2023a). Instead of language: Confusion. Sigmund Freud/Sándor Ferenczi. In: R. Soreanu, J. Staberg, & J. Willner (eds), *Ferenczi Dialogues: On Trauma and Catastrophe* (pp. 23–71). Leuven: Leuven University Press.

Staberg, J. (2023b). Complicated dialogue: Ferenczi (re-)reading Beyond the pleasure principle. *Imago Budapest*, 12(3): 30–42.

Staberg, J. (2024). Ferenczi thinking beyond the pleasure principle. In: H. Westerink, J. Willner, & P. Van Haute (eds), *Towards the Limits of Freudian Thinking: Critical Edition and Readings of Beyond the Pleasure Principle* (pp. 257–283). Leuven: Leuven University Press.

Stewart, H. (2012). Regression post-Ferenczi. In: T. Keve & J. Szekacs-Weisz (eds), *Ferenczi and His World: Rekindling the Spirit of the Budapest School* (pp. 129–137). London: Karnac.

Willner, J. (2023). Catastrophes and genitality: Ferenczi's *Thalassa* and the politics of bioanalysis. In: R. Soreanu, J. Staberg, & J. Willner (eds), *Ferenczi Dialogues: On Trauma and Catastrophe* (pp. 91–130). Leuven: Leuven University Press.

Chapter 1

The Psychic Life of Fragments

On Splitting and Its Times

On Scars, Memory and Symbols

In his *Clinical Diary*, Ferenczi sees '[m]emory [as] a collection of *scars of shocks* in the ego' (Ferenczi, 1932a, p. 111). To have memory means to possess the capacity to be affected, and most of the time this includes being overwhelmed, or broken, or split. Ferenczi (1931c, p. 244) speaks of 'the development of memory from the mental scar-tissue created by bad experiences'. I would like to linger for a moment in the realm of this enigmatic construction – the *scar-tissue*. The scar-tissue is a collection of closed – or partly closed – traumatic wounds that have become connected in a relatively enduring way. The scar-tissue can also be read as the structural effect in the psyche of cumulative attempts at dealing with traumatic wounds, first and foremost in the sense of surviving them. The psyche makes a construction out of the scars, which gives the shape of the ego, and which is also the matter of memory. Seen through the prism of the scar-tissue, trauma is no longer unchanging, immobile and stale, assimilable to a dead space, but it becomes both memory-constructive and ego-constructive.

In my previous work, I argued that 'memory-wounds' are not to be read as 'wounds of memory' or 'wounds to memory' (Soreanu, 2018b). Instead, memory-wounds are those kinds of wounds out of which memory is made. They are 'wounds-toward-memory'. They are the wounds that through particular transformations (closing, partly closing, reopening) can come to form someone's memory – or the 'scar-tissue' that Ferenczi talks about.

Here, I am in resonance with what Avgi Saketopoulou (2023, p. 2) has called 'traumatophilia', which she describes as a 'hospitable attitude to the revisitation of trauma'. Traumatophobia, in her view, is assuming that trauma is a still and dead space. Also, it is assuming that we can rid ourselves of the trauma by fully narrativising it, or healing it, or working

DOI: 10.4324/9781032715926-2

through it. Traumatophobia might also be, I would add, the insistence that we should do away with the term 'trauma', because we have exhausted it and dragged it into incorrect debates. Throughout this chapter, I insist on staying with trauma and also with wounds, scars and scar-tissues.

Proposing a 'traumatophilic touching of wounds', Saketopoulou (2023, p. 134) reminds us that 'wounds never fully close. They leave behind marks and scabs that can reopen and that we are strangely drawn to touch. To touch them, we must first reopen them, which involves cracking open their encasements'. Psychoanalysis is work on wounds. It is a form of endurance across the reopening and re-closing of wounds. Ferenczi too imagines the psychoanalytic process as unfolding around 'wounds':

> Psycho-analysis [...] is a proceeding that seeks to cure neurotic conflict not by a fresh displacement or temporary repression, but radically. It endeavours not to tie up psychic wounds but to lay them bare, to render them conscious.
>
> (Ferenczi, 1908b, p. 29)

Jean Laplanche also defines the psychoanalytic process in relation to wounds. For him, the aim of psychoanalysis is to 'maintain the injury by the other open' ['*maintien de la blessure par l'autre*'] (Laplanche, 1999a, p. 241) and to 'reopen at privileged moments the wound of the unexpected, of the enigma' (Laplanche, 1999b, p. 48; see also Saketopoulou, 2023, p. 133). In all these formulations, we can no longer imagine a resolute closing of a traumatic wound by a process of completed mourning, but a constant movement of getting closer to wounds and re-opening and re-closing them.

Ferenczi's constructions around 'wounds', 'scars' and 'scar-tissues' point to an important quality of the traumatic shock: one of the results of the trauma is precisely the precipitation of representation, of images, of capacities of relating, of specific faculties and even hyper-faculties, and not the interruption of symbolisation. For Ferenczi, this precipitation of the imaginative process happens through the operation of the 'unresting Eros':

> I have no hesitation in regarding even memory-traces as scars, so to speak, of traumatic impressions, i.e. as products of the destructive instinct, which, however, the unresting Eros nevertheless understands how to employ for its own ends, i.e. for the preservation of life. Out of these it shapes a new psychical system, which enables the ego to orientate itself more correctly in its environment, and to form sounder

> judgements. In fact it is only the destructive instinct that 'wills evil', while it is Eros that 'creates good' out of it.
>
> (Ferenczi, 1926)

The traumatic shock is both ego-destructive and ego-constructive. Through the work of the life drive, traumatic impressions can be re-arranged and take the shape of a 'new psychical system'. The ego itself is much more malleable and plastic than we are used to believing, and in certain circumstances the wounds in the scar-tissue that makes up the ego can reopen. In moments of traumatic shock, the ego becomes completely flexible; it loses its solidity, or loses the level of resistance that is needed for it to be a separate psychic agency. The ego can in some cases be entirely 'repressed', which means it is to a large extent pushed back into the id: the result is a psychic system that is made up almost entirely by the id and the superego. In the entry of his *Diary*, on 29 May 1932, Ferenczi writes:

> Fear dissolves the rigidity of the ego (resistance) so completely that the material of the ego becomes as though capable of being moulded *photochemically* – is in fact always moulded – by external stimuli. Instead of my asserting *myself*, the external world (an alien will) asserts itself at my expense; it forces itself upon me and *represses* the ego. (Is this the primal form of 'repression'?)
>
> (Ferenczi, 1932a, p. 11)

The 'photochemical moulding' of the ego is at the heart of having a memory. It is in this sense that memory can be seen as a collection of scars of shocks suffered by the ego. A certain amount of autoplastic reactivity is unavoidable. In this reading, to be wounded is to be in possession of the capacity to be affected. This 'being-affected' is not gentle or gradual: it is sudden and often takes the form of an intrusion or the imposition of an 'alien will' that dissolves or dislodges the ego.

There is an important qualitative demarcation in the field of memory made by Ferenczi, which I have found to be an anchoring companion in the consulting room: he imagines different registers of memory, or different ways of making an inscription in the psyche, or perhaps differently arranged scar-tissues. Memory operates both through the ego and through the id, constituting two regimes or tracks of memory, defined in their difference by their object-relatedness (Stanton, 1991, p. 84). In the *regime of ego memories*, we encounter 'projected sensations', referring to the environment and to external occurrences. These tend to produce effects of objectivity, and they are experienced as verifiable consciously. These kinds of memories can be represented and narrativised, and they can also be subject to processes of repression. In the *regime of id memories*, we find 'bodily sensations', referring to primal life and death trends (*Züge*). When these are elaborated retrospectively by the ego, they are lived as emotions. We can imagine this track of memory as registering affectively charged impressions from the scene of trauma and then returning to them and reviving them, mostly because they are bound up with suffering and a sense of being overwhelmed. These disparate marks cannot be represented consciously or narrativised. They can sometimes fleetingly appear in traumatic dreams or in states of regression.

How are inscriptions made in the register of memories of the id, in the absence of conscious memory, or even thinking processes? The traumatic shock can produce a state of paralysis which is incompatible with any sort of psychic spontaneity or activity of psychic defence. The paralysis is not a fleeting state or a moment of adaptation. Instead, it is capable of changing the structural organisation of the psyche, and it generates 'frozen fragments' of the psyche, which are silent, deadened and de-libidinised. The absolute paralysis of motility in the moment of the attack includes the inhibition of perception and, with it, the inhibition of thinking (Ferenczi, 1931b, p. 240). The traumatic impressions that occur at the time of the attack cannot be recorded via the system of memory of the ego, because this would involve the presence of thinking, even if we are talking about processes of repression. These impressions are thus taken up by the psyche without any sort of resistance. Ferenczi hesitates between suggesting that 'no memory traces of such impressions remain, even in the unconscious, and thus the causes of the trauma cannot be recalled from memory traces' and describing the elements of the new system of memory of the id (idem). In Chapter 2, I will discuss in more detail the precision of the traumatic marks retained in the system of memory of the id. For now, it may be helpful to imagine them as disparate impressions that are collected from the trauma scene, in the first instance incompatible with thoughts, and are presented to the psyche (but cannot be represented).

How does the regime of memory of the id interact with the regime of memory of the ego? Can the emotionality of the bodily sensations and the objectivity-effect of the projected sensations come to be connected? We are here in a position to further qualify the nature of psychoanalytic work: it entails a constant movement between the different registers of memory and their particular modalities of retaining a mark. In the analyst's presence, the analysand weaves ever more connections between the memory of the ego and the memory of the id. This does not mean reconstructing some 'truth' of the scene of trauma, or returning to 'how things really were', but creating new links between the registers in a temporality different from that of the scene of trauma. This type of construction across registers, which involves the analyst, can make the suffering more bearable.

This new situation of memory, organised into two registers, intervenes in how we think of representation, language, symbol and symptom. Ferenczi's formulation resonates with Walter Benjamin's conception of language, underpinned by the idea of *mimesis* between words and things. Language is both physical and psychic. There is an inscription of materiality at the core of every word. This inscription results from the operation of analogy, through which symbols are made. The primary analogies take us back to the body and to the child's act of establishing correspondences between body parts and the external reality. Just as symbols express the body, words imitate things. As Ferenczi writes: 'In its origin, language is imitation, in other words, vocal reproduction of sounds and noises produced by things, or that are produced through them' (Ferenczi, 1913a, p. 228). And later, in his *Clinical Diary*, he adds: 'To speak is to imitate. The gesture and speech (voice) imitate objects of the world around. "Ma-ma" is magic of imitation' (Ferenczi, 1932a, p. 151). Ultimately, Ferenczi sees speech as a form of permanent imitation, which the subject develops so as to tell the story of the trauma:

> a part of the ego remains undestroyed, indeed, it seeks to profit from this demolition (scars). The traumatic *mimicry impressions* are utilised as memory-traces, useful to the ego: 'dog' = bowwow, bowwow. When I am frightened of a dog, I become a dog.
>
> (1932a, pp. 112–113)

To imagine these complicated transubstantiations between body and language, we need elements of a new psychoanalytic vocabulary. One idea that is useful here and deserves our attention is that of 'materialisation'. There is always a potential for materialisations to be available to the psyche, which means that language can convert back to matter or come to 'reference' the body by way of a symptom or another arrangement that is *between* the psyche and the soma. Ferenczi proposes a 'stereochemistry' (1922, p. 369), a spatial model of the various parts of the human organism and their connection with external reality. He speaks of 'transitory symptoms' (Ferenczi, 1912, p. 198) in which emotions are expressed via organic reactions or reorganisations. For instance, emotional bitterness will cause 'a bitter feeling in the tongue' (1912, p. 198). However, as Galina Hristeva stresses, Ferenczi's stereochemistry is not set up to register only dark and painful symptoms. Instead, it is a move to a 'physiology of pleasure', where '[a]esthetics is a product of human physiology, which is determined by complicated associations and links of the organs' (Hristeva, 2013, p. 344). Various parts of the body become connected in intricate, artful, and lively configurations.

It is no wonder that Ferenczi returns to the old image of hysteria, to 'Uterus loquitur' (Ferenczi, 1919a, p. 103), but he gives it a completely novel treatment. The 'speaking uterus' is no poetisation of the anxiety of the theorist in relation to feminine sexuality or female jouissance. Instead, 'Uterus loquitur' is at the centre of a rereading of hysterical materialisation as a form of creativity. As Ferenczi writes:

> [the type of hysterical symptom-formation described] might be called a materialization phenomenon, since its essence consists in the realization of a wish, as though by magic, out of the material in the body at its disposal and – even if in primitive fashion – by a plastic representation, just as an artist moulds the material of his conception or as the occultists imagine the "apport" or the "materialization" of objects at the mere wish of a medium.
>
> (Ferenczi, 1919, p. 96)

Ferenczi takes the analogy between hysteria and making art to its final conclusion. Confronted with a stimulus (often tremendous in its intensity and nature), the organism has two paths of action. One is to modify external reality in such a way that self-destruction and self-reconstruction are unnecessary and that the ego's equilibrium remains unaltered – this path Ferenczi calls 'alloplasty' (1930a, p. 221). The other is to turn the libido inwards and to alter the ego or parts of the ego (by destruction, fragmentation, splitting, reconstruction) – this path he calls 'autoplasty' (1930a).

As he arrived at this metapsychological clarity, the observation of hysterical symptoms functioned as a kind of initial creative 'knot' for Ferenczi. As he puts it:

> Hysteria is, as Freud says, a caricature of art. Hysterical "materializations", however, show us the organism in its entire plasticity, indeed in its preparedness for art. It might prove that the purely "auto-plastic" tricks of the hysteric are prototypes, not only for the bodily performances of "artists" and actors, but also for the work of those creative artists who no longer manipulate their own bodies but material from the external world.
>
> (Ferenczi, 1919, p. 104)

This superposing of the grammar of the alloplastic act (construction/destruction on the outside) with the grammar of the autoplastic act (construction/destruction on the inside) thus goes far beyond the recognition of the creativity of the hysterical symptom. It formulates a new answer to the problem of connection between psyche and soma, which includes constructions, harmonisations and fragmentations, in ways that involve an entire mesh of organs, tissues, cells, fluids and neuronal circuits.

As Cornelius Castoriadis (1987) showed, one of the distinguishing characteristics of the human psyche is the intricate relationship between representational pleasure and organ pleasure. Castoriadis (1989a, p. 380) argues that the psyche does not merely 'represent' the body but instead 'duplicates' it: '[t]he body, (more exactly, the "actions/passions" of the body) is source of pleasure, but this pleasure has to be "doubled" by representation'. In other words, to invent languages and to invent relations between words, body parts, organs and other forms of matter is a fundamental source of pleasure.

Ferenczi introduces a new and much-needed vocabulary around pleasure: he talks about various kinds of pleasure, which in my view he treats as expressions of a plurality of drives. Five years before Freud introduced the opposition between the life drive and the death drive in his 1920 text 'Beyond the Pleasure Principle', Ferenczi spoke, in his paper 'The Analysis of Comparisons' (1915, p. 406), of the 'pleasure of resemblance' [*Lust an der Ähnlichkeit*]; the 'pleasure in repetition' [*Wiederholungslust*]; and the 'pleasure in rediscovery' [*Wiederfindungslust*]. This composes a non-dualistic picture of the drives. Repetition is here not bound with anxiety and with the death drive, as it appears in Freud's famous 1920 formulation on repetition-compulsion; it is instead bound with Ferenczi's philosophical and clinical idea of imitation, where any kind of psychic growth or creativity involves a certain degree of mimetism. Anticipating his later ideas on projection/introjection, Ferenczi (1915, p. 407) writes: 'The tendency to rediscover what is loved in all the things of the hostile outer world is also probably the primitive source of symbolism'.

Clinically, the 'pleasure of resemblance' [*Lust an der Ähnlichkeit*] refers primarily to a 'venturing out' of the body by way of observing similarities between body parts and things and between sets of closer or more distant things. The 'pleasure in repetition' [*Wiederholungslust*] refers to a kind of repetition that is not connected to the death drive via compulsion, but it has to do with 'settling into' the relationship between the ego and the environment and also into walking the distance between body parts and the things of the world, including other living beings. The 'pleasure of rediscovery' [*Wiederfindungslust*] marks a temporal syncope, where an object (or a comparison) is set aside for a while, only to be later on joyfully picked up where it was left off.

To Ferenczi's vocabulary on pleasure, I add the *pleasure of analogy*. This might be understood as closely related to the 'pleasure of resemblance' [*Lust an der Ähnlichkeit*] (Ferenczi, 1915, p. 406), but it is meant to render it more radically relational by insisting on the fact that the 'things' that constitute the objects of the pleasure of analogy are *relations*. The pleasure of analogy is the doubly relational pleasure: *the pleasure of establishing a relation between two relations*. The pleasure of analogy is the libidinal ground of the social bond exceeding the Oedipal configuration. For the pleasure of analogy to be felt, three elements are not sufficient; there will need to be at least four, five, or potentially more. The simplest grammar of the pleasure of analogy, involving four presences, is: 'What X is to me, Y is to Z'.

Ferenczi reminds us of the 'principle of harmony' which makes mutuality possible. In this mutuality, there is 'simultaneous giving and taking' that renders the life of the 'ego' possible and bearable. What interests us here are artful compositions and linkings which include cells, organs, body membranes, but also the body of the other, inorganic material and substances. Psychoanalyst Radmila Zygouris (1999), in her book *Pulsões de Vida*, coins a new term pertaining to the sphere of Eros: *aimance*. Aimance results from a condensation of the French words *aimer* [to love] and *aimant* [magnet]. Zygouris alerts us to the fact that being affected by a common object opens a field of intensities between two (or more) people, leading to an intensification of Eros. As she puts it, '[t]he fields of aimance are collective' (1999). She is imagining a libidinised and magnetic social sphere, traversed by shared modes of being affected. Indeed, being able to be affected is the psychoanalyst's main 'tool'.

In these pages, I would like to take the reader into the realm of a psychoanalysis of scars, wounds and scar-tissues. But while being attentive to scars, I also aim to extend our understanding of relational pleasures. Not only the pleasure of establishing a relationship between objects (linking), nor only the pleasure of being affected by a common object (aimance), but the pleasure of discovering the analogies that are involved in investing in a common object. This pleasure of analogy follows the grammar: 'I stand in relation to an object, in the same way that you stand in relation to an object'.

Vignette: On Learning a Word

Tia arrived in my consulting room ridden with noisy symptoms. She had a kind of insomnia that prevented her from going into profound and restful states of sleep, and she was feeling she had not been able to sleep properly in five years. She had very frequent panic attacks that had become so severe that on many days she could not get out of the house at all; she could not get on a bus or in an elevator. Apart from this, she displayed in the analysis a great number of 'transitory symptoms' (as Ferenczi calls them) of a hysterical grammar, such as feeling pins and needles in her arms; frequent headaches and migraines; and feeling 'pain attacks' in different parts of her body. At the intersection of the many symptoms, the beginning of the analysis had a certain hallucinatory quality. It seems that this conjunction of symptoms was transporting us into another world, one with its own rules of gravity and its own relations between space, time and bodies.

Tia is 46 years of age. Her mother is Afro-Brazilian, while her father is White. This detail will prove very important, as Tia was successful in performing a kind of whitening of her skin from the inside out. In wishing to appear White, it is as if she has successfully 'hidden' away her mother, blocking her from her physical appearance, partly in an attempt to achieve separation. Tia and I do not share a mother tongue; the analysis unfolds in Portuguese, which is her mother tongue, but not mine.

After the first few months of the analysis, I was troubled to find out that Tia suffered from bulimia. She had been throwing up every day for five years. One of her most used words was 'nojo' – 'nausea' – and the descriptions of her experience included a great number of references to swallowing whole, being swallowed, swallowing one's feelings.

A few months into the analysis, Tia had a very powerful episode of remembrance of a time in her early adolescence, when she was being persecuted by both her mother and her three sisters for her different appearance. She was tall, thin and light-skinned, while they were all shorter and dark-skinned. On one day, while she was walking down the road alone, her older sister, who was near the road with a group of friends, shouted at her: 'Pau-de-vira-tripa!'.

As she was telling me this episode, Tia stopped and asked me: 'Do you know what "pau-de-vira-tripa" means?' I answered: 'No, I have not heard this expression before, but I imagine what it might mean. Would you like to tell me what it means?' Tia explained that it referred to a wooden stick that is used to turn the intestines of sacrificed animals inside out before they are dried.

In this moment, I learned a new word from Tia. The analytic pair does not share the mother tongue, but the word that is taught/learnt holds the key to a symptom and enables a chain of re-translations, where the foreignness of the original giving-of-a-name and the subject's solitude and exile in this name are captured. Curiously, it is an analyst's missing word that is implicated in making sense of a symptom.

After that day and into her adolescence, 'pau-de-vira-tripa' remained one of her humiliating denominations. I felt that this episode had an extremely important charge. I repeated the expression to her several times. It became our focus, in that session and over the next few months of the analysis. I directed her to the *verb* inside the expression. Together, we imagined the movement: it is a movement of an intestine being turned inside out, over and over again. Like it is the case when she throws up. It is also an instrument that is used on a sacrificed animal.

These interventions became aligned with another set of interpretations following her description of phone conversations with her mother, whom she had not seen in person for a very long time: in these conversations, she felt an invisible thread of vitality, or energy, or liquid, going out from her in the direction of her mother. She would tell me, 'I am feeling depleted'. But she would not be able to stop the cycles of depletion. I interpreted this as her feeling a kind of inversion of the direction of the mother's milk. Instead of milk flowing into her, as a child, she was feeling that the milk was flowing out of her, as her mother was resentful of her daughters and found any aspect of their care a burden and an inconvenience. At the intersection of these two sets of interpretations, her bulimia gradually cleared out in a few weeks' time. Surely, the background feeling of depletion, of being emptied out by an external overpowering presence, of being robbed of her insides, was much more difficult to address than the symptom that emerged from it. Only recently, Tia has become more able to hold on to her things and not feel compelled to give them up. This symptom was very important, like a 'knot' of the entire process.

Over the years, we moved from concerns of fusion and devouring, where many things were swallowed and/or vomited, to preoccupations with what is retained and what is given. Towards the end of the analysis, the preoccupations moved to the pleasure of experience, to experimenting, to finding a house, to connecting to her environment, and to feeling more at home in the world.

*

But let us stay with the word.
The word we stumbled across was also a thing.
Pressing into our bodies.
Pressing on the transference, or wrapped in the other things we were passing between us.

So what were we doing, us two, patient and analyst, how were we being across this word? We were passing a wooden stick, a magic stick, from the couch to the chair and from the chair to the couch.

I try not to drop it.
I try to give it back without moves that are too sudden.
Pau-de-vira-tripa.
In my mind, it is all hyphenated.
Like the names of some fairly-tale creatures, endowed with special powers.

Analysis means removing the hyphens, one by one, to release the verb.
The verb is 'virar'. To veer. To turn inside out. To turn upside down.
The verb is in a series with the bulimic symptom.

Tia was estranged in her own language.
Analysis, here, took the place that Russian formalist Victor Shklovsky assigned to art – as he writes: 'art exists [so] that one may recover the sensation of life; it exists to make one feel things, to make the stony *stony*.'

So I would say: to make the wooden, *wooden*.
The tragic wood can return to itself, after it has made a detour through an other.
An other who is short of one word.
A foreigner who is short of one word.

Pau-de-vira-tripa brought me and Tia into the 'fire of tongues', as Julia Kristeva would put it, an exit from representation; and also into the midst of the fact that language contains the potential for its own renewal.

To let the word do its work, what was needed was to allow the transmutation of the word into the body and of the body into the word. This is similar to what borderline patients experience, a kind of confusion between the space of the body and the space of the word. Julia Kristeva reminds us about this approximation between the borderline experience and the experience of poetic language – again, the 'fire of tongues'.

And so, to repeat the 'pau-de-vira-tripa', to pass it across the space between patient and analyst, perhaps until its hyphens lift, becomes a sort of incantation. It is a repetition that is not in direct connection to the death drive, but indeed a reconstructive repetition. Within this sort of repetition, language itself suffers a transmutation, like in one of Vicente Huidobro's (2003) poems: '*Now I'm rosebush and speak in rosebush language/ And I say/ Rise rose rorosarose/ Rise rose to the day/ Rose ary arose to the sun*'.

*

Tia was unhomely in her world,
because she was unhomely in her word, 'pau-de-vira-tripa'.
In the word that was called upon her.

In the word that she was called into.

In the word that she was confused by.

The purpose of the analysis was to make this word vibrate oneirically, reviving its lost memories and associations.

*

'Pau-de-vira-tripa' was thus a powerful word.
The kind of word that makes the gut turn, so as to follow the mandate of the verb.
So might we say that there was a complicated analogy between the word and the gut?
And that working on the verb produced direct effects in the gut?

In a 1921 essay, Ferenczi writes: '[T]he symbol – a thing of flesh and blood' (Ferenczi, 1921, p. 352). How does free-association alter flesh and matter? There is no magic way in which this occurs, but it is a possibility that is inscribed in the development of what Ferenczi calls 'the sense of reality'. In a distinct stage of the development of the sense of reality – the stage of the 'gesture-language' – the main activity of the child is that of establishing correspondences between her own body and the outside world. In fact, as Ferenczi writes, '[o]n the one hand, the child in this stage sees in the world nothing but images of [her] corporeality, on the other [she] learns to represent by means of [her] body the whole multifariousness of the outer world' (Ferenczi, 1913a, p. 228). Thus, the 'symbolic' is grounded in the stage of the 'gesture-language', during which strong connections are established, with enduring effects throughout life, between the body and that which lies beyond it. Here, Ferenczi comes close to thinkers such as Julia Kristeva (1984, 2000), Félix Guattari (2011), Cornelius Castoriadis (1987) and especially José Gil (1997), a perhaps lesser-known Portuguese philosopher.

José Gil (1997, p. 23) speaks of the 'fluctuating signifier', which is an energy, a force that is impossible to signify across codes. Here, the 'permutator of codes' is the body (1997). The semantic units are the gestural units. Affect is the global modulator that integrates a multiplicity of units in an individuated sequence.

It is crucial to mark the way Ferenczi differentiates 'unsubstantial allegory' from 'the symbol'. Not every analogy is symbolic in a psychoanalytic sense. The symbol emerges from a particular kind of affectively charged non-arbitrariness. How so? First, the symbol has a physiological basis: it 'expresses in some ways the whole body or its functions' (Ferenczi, 1921, p. 355). Second, one of the two terms that make up a symbolic analogy (they can be either things or ideas) is invested in consciousness with an inexplicable overcharge of affect. This surplus of affect is rooted in the unconscious identification with another thing/idea. The overcharge of affect is thus displaced from one thing/idea to another. When Ferenczi distinguishes between unsubstantial analogy and symbolic analogy, he contrasts the bi-dimensionality of the first with the three-dimensionality of the second. But what is the third dimension that he is referring to?

I argue that the 'third dimension' is the analogy-work of the mind/body of the analyst, linking the two series of elements that bear a homology (while having one of the series invested with inexplicable affect). The psychoanalyst thus works with symbols that are things 'of flesh and blood'.

By not knowing the expression 'pau-de-vira-tripa', I was perhaps more struck by its materiality, by its being gut-bound, and by the movement prescribed by its verb.

*

In our work together, Tia and I were on the painful rim of blackness. I was on the whiteness side of the rim, and she was on the blackness side. Entangled in our difference, we were able to work out that she had always been too White for her family, for her own kind. But later on, she was always too Black for any other 'kind', indeed for the 'kind' she attributed to me.

One year into the analysis, it was revealed that one of the most important fantasies that had a sustaining role for the analysis was that *I was unlike anyone else she has ever met.* I was not from there, with a strange accent and with unusual manners. I was a foreigner from a far-off land.

I will trace the transformation of this fantasy and its function in the analysis. About one year into the analysis, Tia became able to speak about this fantasy and even interpret it herself. She recognised the fact that what she needed from me in the initial stage was to be able to place me as very 'far-off', or untouched by the things and events that were a part of her infantile world, and which she saw as *abject*. What she had done with her previous therapists (who shared her mother tongue) was precisely to place them *within the abjection* and therefore reject them and feel rejected by them. My function was to 'embody' the difference, so that only later she could become able to 'symbolise' the difference. My role was to not be 'part of the same misery' (as she used to say), and thus to be a kind of incipient, emergent, and concretised 'outside'. A place/person that has 'nothing to do' with her childhood.

Two years into the analysis, she remembered some Polish Jewish women from her neighbourhood, whom she liked very much, and she started to find some resemblances between them and me. I was starting to move positions myself in her fantasy; I was less needed as something she had 'never seen before' and more an object used for the integration of the not very numerous good memories she had from her childhood.

In the beginning of the analysis, Tia had a very vivid transferential dream. The analyst was having sex with a dark-skinned man while Tia was nowhere, an immaterial observer, blended into the environment. This primal scene was a racialised encounter. When she started her analysis, Tia was overt in her statements of hatred and disgust in relation to all things that had to do with negritude and with her Afro-Brazilian heritage.

For many years, this dream returned as a 'knot' in her analysis. The more we dealt with the enigmatic aspects of this love encounter, the more her hatred of blackness was transformed. Instead of hatred, what emerged were many images that placed us in 'the wake' (to use Christina Sharpe's words) of slavery, in slavery's afterlives (Sharpe, 2016). She was able to speak about a kind of violence that she had not caused, but in which she was entangled through being Black. What is important here is that race appeared in the psyche as sexualised. Working on this racialised primal scene allowed Tia to experience a state of curiosity, fascination and even love in relation to Afro-Brazilian culture and religion. She reflected on various cultural and religious symbols, which she started seeing as her own.

My not speaking a particular word (and perhaps several words, over the years) was, I believe, part of what made such dreams dreamable, and also part of what allowed me to interpret them in a way that is bound up with a change of psychosexual positions. Strangely, the event of Tia putting a word in my mouth created a solid bodily connection, which was not oblivious to the violence of the colonial encounter, or to the rim of blackness, on which we were differently positioned. And so, at this time, after Tia's analysis has ended, I am thinking of Oswaldo de Andrade, who writes: 'Only Anthropophagy unite us. Socially. Economically. Philosophically'. Or, differently put: what unites us is an ancestral time in which we would have eaten each other's bodies and thus each other's words.

*

We know that Freud used the cannibal trope in a conservative manner to emphasise the gap between the primitive and the civilised (Freud, 1913; Vyrgioti, 2021). In post-Freudian writers, there are terms that do not name the cannibal in the room but do allude to it or invoke it by references to devouring, ingesting, ingurgitating, eating up, swallowing up, but also introjecting, incorporating – this is the case in object-relations writing. Some of these indirect references to the cannibal figure often end up with the same conservative polarity between the primitive and the civilised. But I believe there are some radical possibilities in the cannibal trope and also in critically questioning and decolonising a series of key psychoanalytic terms that bear the hidden cannibal reference.

What do we learn if we become invested in an alternative set of curious terms around regurgitating, extrojection and ex-corporation? This investment is a gesture of a psychoanalytic theory in the aftermath of cannibalism. The fantasy of regurgitating, of the psychic reversal of an introjection, is one of great importance. By following it, we can ask: what does regurgitating do to the racist matrix?

This interest in a new series of terms around regurgitation cuts across the distinction proposed in 1961 by Lévi-Strauss in his work *Tristes Tropiques*, differentiating between anthropophagic societies, which in a sense 'eat up' and assimilate foreigners and foreignness; and anthropoemic societies [from the Greek word *emein*, to vomit] where the foreigner is expulsed, segregated, or isolated (Lévi-Strauss, 1961). In the first case we are dealing with the violence of inclusion and in the second with the violence of exclusion. What I am interested in is a third form, a non-violent vomiting, where regurgitation creates something new and valuable.

The gut is a political place (Wilson, 2015). Among psychoanalytic thinkers, Ferenczi is particularly observant of the creativity of organs, and he stays close to the question, 'what does an organ do?' His understanding of hysteria is a radically reconfigured one, in the sense that it has a complex way of discussing the creativities of the hysterical symptom. In his own writings on hysteria, Ferenczi is less interested in coughs and paralyses and more fascinated by the mobilisation of the 'inside' of bodies in a phenomenon that he calls 'hysterical materialisation' (Ferenczi, 1919). Discussing the globus hystericus (a lump in the throat), he descends into the digestive tract and becomes interested in the material transformations that take place in the patients' throats:

> The patients themselves speak of a lump stuck in their throats, and we have every reason to believe that the corresponding contractions of the circular and longitudinal musculature of the oesophagus produce not only the paraesthesia of a foreign body, but that a kind of foreign body, a lump, really is brought about.
>
> (Ferenczi, 1919, p. 92)

The accent here is on the productive and materialising force of hysteria: the lump in the throat is not merely a hallucination but part of a new 'grammar' of organs, a stirring up of the tissues of the throat, or of the contents of the stomach, or of the intestinal matter, which implies a capacity for condensation, displacement, repetition, or identification. This showcasing of the creativities of the hysterical symptom has important implications for how we can imagine the relationship between the psyche and the soma. In short, there is a 'horizontalising' gesture here, where the soma is just as capable of complex acts as the psyche.

The bulimic symptom, by imitating the matter of the word 'pau-de-vira-tripa', was pointing to the violence of the racist matrix. In this case, it was pointing to the violence of mixed heritage, where the subject's exile of the skin proclaims: 'I am both too White and too Black'. There was thus value in the patient's fantasy of regurgitating and even in her enacting this fantasy. This bulimic symptom was the route to an important scene of racial suffering. It was part of the reversal of a violent introjection, the extrojection of the impossible statement: 'You are always both too White and too Black'.

The Psychic Life of Fragments

Psychic Fragments Have a Life

It is no small task to imagine how psychic splitting happens and what is the life of the fragments resulting from the splitting. I would say it takes a radical expansion of the clinical imagination. The clinic of our times is traversed by references to a range of 'dissociative' processes and forms of splitting and fragmentation, but these processes often remain enigmatic and underspecified. I argue that Ferenczi offers a key revision to the work of Sigmund Freud. To a far greater extent than Freud, Ferenczi centred his psychoanalytic thought around trauma, focusing on how the traumatic shock leads to radical forms of psychic splitting. Ferenczi thinks of these processes in terms of complex defence mechanisms, and even the formation of new psychic agencies, which we can only understand if we envision the various fragments resulting from splitting as having a psychic 'life' of their own. In his *Clinical Diary*, written during the last year of his life in 1932, he outlines a *metapsychology of fragmented psyches* (Soreanu, 2018b) against the backdrop of both personal and political catastrophes (Soreanu et al., 2023). The form of the diary is itself fragmented: it presents an unfinished theory, containing clinical observations and metapsychological constructions in which Ferenczi draws from his work with severely traumatised patients. His core idea is that, given the enormity of suffering experienced during the traumatic attack, psychic survival would have been impossible without radically splitting into fragments (Soreanu et al., 2023).

For Ferenczi, psychic fragmentation is the ubiquitous operation of the psyche. To approach the 'culture of fragments' that is the result of psychic trauma, however, we need to unpack Ferenczi's unique vocabulary of fragmentation, which includes references to fractures, splits, atomisations, pulverisations, leakages, detritus, but also new formations, protective membranes, expansions, contagions, and inner growths.

As I showed in the previous section, Ferenczi reconfigures the relationship between the psyche and the soma, and he brings us to a kind of hyphenated psycho-soma, where even the hysterical symptom is susceptible to being a form of creativity, unfolding in its own language. With Ferenczi, we are attentive to forms of radical plasticity, to surprising modes of psychic splitting that result from the scene of trauma, to 'semifluid' bodies and organs that reshape, retract, and grow new curious parts. What does it mean, in today's clinic, to follow Ferenczi's pathos for transformation? What does it mean to think, to write, and to practise clinically at the limits of what we can imagine for bodies and what bodies can imagine for themselves?[1]

Being animated by these questions means addressing the 'phenomenological gap' in psychoanalysis around the problem of psychic splitting.

There is a deficit of *precise* descriptions about *what is being split in the psyche; about the process of splitting; and about the psychic life of the fragments that result from the splitting* (Soreanu, 2018a, Soreanu et al., 2023). Not all of these fragments map on to the three Freudian agencies: id, ego and superego. There are kinds of splitting that make demands on us and that point to a need for metapsychological revision. I believe that Ferenczi addresses this phenomenological gap by articulating a metapsychology of fragmented psyches. In his work, we find a series of original and very precise formulations on splitting.

Ferenczi invites us to creatively engage the following questions: what is the 'stuff' that the psyche is splitting? Is it the ego? Is it the self on the whole (including the ego, but also other agencies)? Is it a part of the ego where a particular introjection happened? Or is it even a part of the ego that an other has successfully projected something onto? (Soreanu, 2018a).

In my previous work (Soreanu, 2018a), I argued that one of Ferenczi's innovations is that he takes us beyond a 'mundane' kind of splitting between the good object and the bad object, and he steps into the terrain of an 'eventful' splitting, a splitting not by the ego but *of* the ego. This eventful kind of splitting results in de-libidinised and re-libidinised stable fragments of the psyche. Indeed, a new psychic structure is formed. We are then confronted with a 'culture of fragments' or with a mosaic of dead parts and alive parts of the psyche. They are fragments that stand in particular kinds of dynamic, economic, and topical relations with one another. In some cases, their relations are so stable, enduring, and structured that they can be seen as relations between agencies of the psyche or inter-systemic relations. We can consider, for instance, the relations between the fragment (or psychic agency) Orpha and the superego, which can work to enhance persecutory demands from the ego. I will turn to this in Chapter 3 of the book.

One important way to trace the psychic life of fragments is to pay attention to their *times*. Some fragments live in an eternal, triumphant present that makes any sequence of acts unimaginable and extracts the subject from any sense of historicity. To a large extent, this book is an exploration of the psychic times of fragments, as experienced in the psychoanalytic consulting room. Following the times of fragments, we can get into the atmosphere of their lives, understood psychoanalytically as dynamic, economic and topographic stories.

The idea of splitting [*Spaltung*] is already present in Freud's work. However, I believe there is an unfinished project in Freud around processes of splitting. On the problem of fragmentation, we can follow Freud in three important directions. Firstly, there is the fundamental splitting that leads to the separation of the psychic agencies (id, ego and superego). This leads Freud to theorise repression. The ego is formed through a particular kind of splitting from the id; while the superego results from further splitting of the ego, seen as an inheritor of the Oedipus complex. Secondly, there is the splitting of representations [*Objektspaltung*], which is given special attention later on by Melanie Klein, with her interest on the splitting between the good object and the bad object. Thirdly, there is the splitting of the ego [*Spaltung* or *Ichspaltung*], explored by Freud in his text 'Splitting of the Ego in the Process of Defence' (Freud, 1938). Here, Freud uses the term to denote a very specific phenomenon which he deems to be at work above all in fetishism and in the psychoses: the co-existence at the heart of the ego of two psychical attitudes towards external reality, in so far as it stands in the way of an instinctual demand. The first of these attitudes takes reality into consideration, while the second disavows it and replaces it with a product of desire. The two attitudes persist side by side without influencing each other. We can understand this persistence as disavowal [*Verleugnung*]. We can consider that this splitting is not strictly an ego defence but a co-existence of two modes of defence. While this third understanding of splitting undoubtedly has profound clinical and theoretical ramifications, I believe that the Freudian project on splitting is unfinished or perhaps too narrowly imagined. We are left with a situation where the splitting of the ego is tied to fetishism, and we do not get very far in terms of engaging the questions I considered above: what is the stuff that the psyche is splitting? And: what are the stable results of processes of fragmentation?

To the Freudian vocabulary on splitting [*spaltung*], Ferenczi brings a qualitative difference: a new register of terms, which I believe constitute his unique mark: he talks of atomisations, pulverisations, and shattering of psychic matter into particles without form. I have discussed this as a process of psychic de-materialisation (Soreanu, 2018a). I include below a multilingual mapping of his terms on splitting, as they appear in the text on the confusion of tongues, a core text in terms of his intervention on fragmentation (Ferenczi, 1933). I included several languages in this mapping (from German and Hungarian, to English, French, Portuguese and Spanish), so as to enable reflection on the reception of Ferenczi's vocabulary on splitting across different psychoanalytic cultures. The past two decades have brought an international 'Ferenczi revival' and, while I here don't insist on this, it is interesting to note how distance from the Freudian terms was engrained in different translations. Ferenczi's 'qualitative difference' appears in the second part of the table, which contains references to splitting into different personalities and also, importantly, to a novel process that does not appear in Freud: atomisation.

The encounter of the subject with the Other is at the heart of Ferenczi's theory of subjectivation. The consequences of this encounter are catastrophic, in the sense of a subversion of the order of things, which is neither only destructive nor only creative. (Etymologically, the term 'catastrophe' is derived from the Greek *καταστροφή*, a sudden turn, but also a conclusion.) In his account of fragmentation, Ferenczi tells a story of both partial

English	**German**	**Hungarian**	**French**	**Portuguese**	**Spanish**
Splitting of the personality (p. 227)	Spaltung der Persönlichkeit (p. 9)	Személyiség hasadás (p. 219)	Clivage de la personnalité (p. 40)	Clivagem da personalidade (p. 115)	División de la personalidad (p. 143)
Splits (p. 227)	Spaltung (p. 9)	Hasadás (p. 219)	Clivage (p. 40)	Clivagem (p. 115)	División (p. 143)
Splitting of the mind (p. 227)	Psychischen Spaltung (p. 9)	Lelki meghasadás (p. 219)	Clivage psychique (p. 40)	Clivagem psíquica (p. 115)	Ruptura psíquica (p. 143)
Split (p. 228)	Gespalten (p. 11)	Meghasadás (p. 221)	Clivé (p. 45)	Dividido (p. 117)	Dividido (p. 145)
Splitting of the personality (p. 229)	Persönlichkeitsspaltung (p. 13)	Személyiséghasadás (p. 223)	Clivage de la personnalité (p. 49)	Fragmentos clivados (p. 120)	División de la personalidad (p. 147)
Fragments (p. 229)	Fragmenten (p. 14)	Töredékek (p. 224)	Fragments, qui se comportent tous comme des personnalités distinctes (p. 51)	Fragmentos que se comportam como personalidades distintas (p. 120)	Personalidades distintas (p. 148)
Fragmentation (p. 229)	Fragmentierung (p. 14)	Fragmentálódás (p. 224)	Fragmentation (p. 51)	Fragmentação (p. 120)	Fragmentación (p. 148)
Atomization (p. 229)	Atomisierung (p. 14)	Atomizálódás (p. 224)	Atomisation (p. 51)	Atomização (p. 120)	Atomización (p. 148)
Ferenczi, S. (1933). The confusion of tongues between adults and the child. In: *Final Contributions to the Problems and Methods of Psycho-analysis*. London: Karnac, 1994.	Ferenczi, S. (1932). Sprachverwirrung zwischen den Erwachsenen und dem Kind. *Internationale Zeitschrift für Psychoanalyse*, 19: 5-15.	Ferenczi S. (1932). Nyelvzavar a felnőttek és a gyermek között. In: B. Buda (Ed.) *A pszichoanalízis és modern irányzatai* (pp. 215-228). Budapest: Gondolat, 1971.	Ferenczi, S. (1932). Confusion de langue entre les adultes et l'enfant. Le langage de la tendresse et de la passion. In: *Psychanalyse. Œuvres complètes, Vol. 4*. Paris: Payot, 1982.	Ferenczi, S. (1932). Confusão de língua entre os adultos e a criança: a linguagem da ternura e da paixão. In: *Obras completes. Psicanálise, Vol, 4*. São Paulo: Martins Fontes Editora, 1992.	Ferenczi, S. (1932). Confusión de lengua entre los adultos y el niño. *Obras completes, Vol. 4* (pp. 139-149). Buenos Aires, Argentina: Amorrortu, 1984.

Figure 1.1 Multilingual Map of Ferenczi's Vocabulary of 'Fragmentation' in *Confusion of Tongues between the Adults and the Child* (1933).

psychic death and of partial survival, as well as the story of the multiplication of forms of psychic life (Soreanu et al., 2023). His work contributes to pluralising the understanding of catastrophe. Surviving the trauma is in itself a tragic outcome: it involves preserving some parts of the psyche, radically transforming others, and severing some other ones. In a conversation with Giselle Galdi, a psychoanalyst and author who has a lifelong engagement with Ferenczi's trauma theory, she qualified the affective atmosphere of his theory as 'tragic optimism'. I agree with this colouring of affect: Ferenczi helps us to understand forms of survival beyond restorative illusions (Soreanu et at, 2023). There is no celebration of fragmentation, but there is also no traumatophobia, no assimilation of the aftermath of trauma to a stale or deadened spate.

In his short piece 'On Shock', Ferenczi (1932b) creates an important image to register this new catastrophic kind of fragmentation, which involves a process akin to one of de-materialisation. As he writes:

> Shock – annihilation of self-regard – of the ability to put up a resistance, and to act and think in defence of one's own self; perhaps even the *organs* which secure self-preservation give up their function or reduce it to a minimum. (The word *Erschütterung* is derived from *schütten*, i.e. to become 'unfest, unsolid', to lose one's own form and to adopt easily and without resistance, an imposed form – 'like a sack of flour').
>
> (Ferenczi, 1932b, pp. 253–254)

The implication is that psychic fragments have lives of their own. This means, for instance, that they are characterised by different temporalities of the psyche, and they also have singular dynamic relations with other fragments. The more we learn about how their difference is lived and how to qualify their difference as analysts – the more we can address the suffering of our patients. Psychic de-materialisation is a particular 'moment' related to the strain that the subject goes through in the scene of trauma, which puts the conscious ego in suspension, indeed abolishes it, while also instilling a sense of being 'outside time', or in an 'eternal present', where there is no sequence, no past, and no future.

One might legitimately ask: why fragmentation? Why does the psyche respond to the pressure of the traumatic attack by splitting? At first, the psyche responds to being overwhelmed by an other by trying to maintain its existing equilibrium and its organisation unchanged. It 'pushes back' against the external stimulus, attempting to modify the external reality (alloplastic adaptation). A necessary condition for this course of psychic action is a highly developed sense of reality. However, if the state of being overwhelmed continues or intensifies – or indeed if the sense of reality is not strong enough – the psyche 'gives up' and turns to self-destruction and self-reconstruction (Ferenczi, 1930a, p. 221). Fragmentation is therefore to be understood as a clever adaptation. Ferenczi (1930d, p. 230) makes clear that fragmentation is an economically advantageous solution to the state of being overwhelmed in the scene of trauma. Firstly, it creates a more 'extended surface' (1930d) towards the external world, making it easier to discharge intense affects. Secondly, fragmentation is a form of giving up 'unified perception' – in a sense, it produces a necessary 'distribution' of pain across segments and fragments. As Ferenczi stresses, '[t]he single fragments suffer for themselves; the unbearable unification of all pain qualities and quantities does not take place' (1930d). Thirdly, by avoiding integration and the interrelation of pain qualities and quantities, the fragments are more pliable, plastic and adaptable. They can further alter themselves and create new growths and even new ad hoc organs. Ferenczi's keen attention to fragments can also be read in his cultural context and by reference to modernism. Ferenczi followed the artistic avant-garde of his time with great interest. In Budapest, he was part of a vibrant intellectual network, which included composers such as Béla Bartók and Zoltán Kodály, and writers such as Sándor Márai (Soreanu et al., 2023). The fragment – as opposed to the 'wholeness' of a composition, imagined to have a beginning, an end, and also an organising principle holding it together – became one of the calling cards of the modernist movement. The fragment was a recognisable, sometimes enigmatic means of creating impact and communicating a message, a 'device' that disturbed conventional notions of space and time in artistic expression. The fragment corresponded to a new sense of the world or sensibility that began to emerge as the nineteenth century ended.

A short excerpt from Pablo Picasso, in a 1945 interview with André Warnod, captures very well this sensibility of fragments, which would have been part of forming Ferenczi's clinical ear. I return to this excerpt often, in teaching Ferenczi's theory of fragments, and I treat it akin to a dream or as the narration of a psychic voice that is arranging the fragments in the scene of trauma. Some get thrown away, while others get reclaimed and rearranged in a meaningful and even artful composition:

> You remember that bull's head I exhibited recently? Out of the handle bars and bicycle seat I made a bull's head which everybody recognized as a bull's head. Thus a metamorphosis was completed: and now I would like to see another metamorphosis take place in the opposite direction. Suppose my bull's head is thrown on the scrap heap. Perhaps one day a fellow will come along and say: 'Why there's something that would come in very handy for the handle bars of my bicycle...' And so a double metamorphosis would have been achieved.
>
> (Picasso, 1945)

There is also a plasticity of fragments or a reversibility of psychic processes that we can imagine while reading this excerpt: what was deadened and de-libidinised can become revivified again, while what was lively can be severed and discarded. And the cycle can begin again.

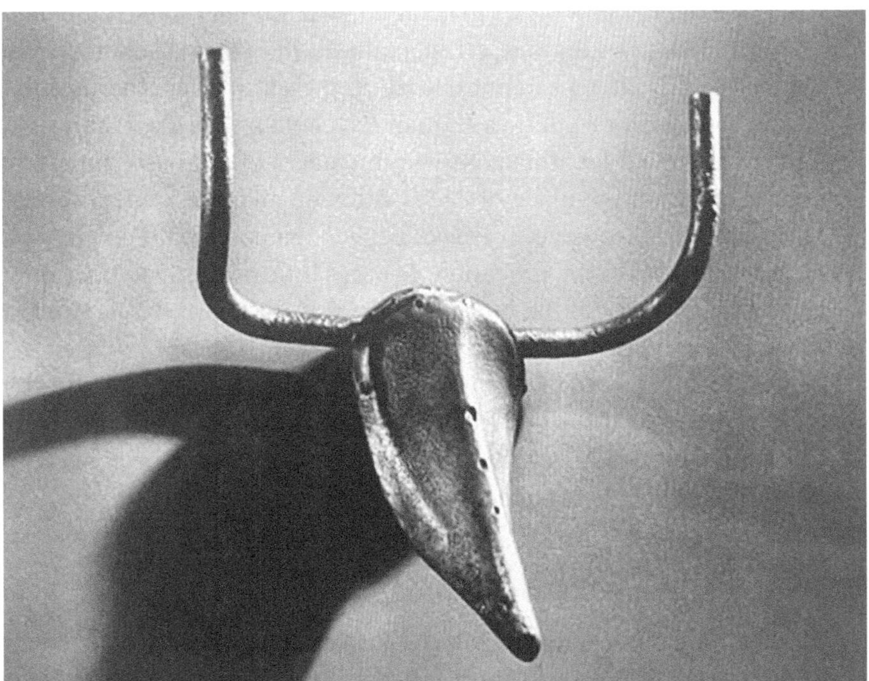

Figure 1.2 'Bull's Head' by Pablo Picasso (1945).

Photograph by the Author.

The Eventful Life of Psychic Fragments

There is a widespread view that the problem of psychic splitting is indissolubly linked to that of identification or that *psychic splitting occurs alongside one aspect or another of the processes of identification.* In Freud there is an important bias towards Oedipal and post-Oedipal identification. Although Freud (1913) refers to more primary and cannibalistic forms of identification (pre-Oedipal), there is no description that can help us make sense of the pre-Oedipal identification processually, which would mean an understanding of the psychic 'moves' through which an object is 'cannibalised'.

In 1913, Freud made the link between identification and eating the person one wishes to be like (Freud, 1913). The reference here was the religious practices of primitive societies. In 1915, while proposing a pregenital sexual drive organisation, Freud introduced a drive-derivative wish/fantasy of early life, 'incorporation of the object', as a model for identification (Freud, 1915, p. 138). Most often, identification is discussed by Freud as a mental process of general importance later in development: a kind of thinking, putting oneself mentally in the place of another. The motivation for this attempt to put oneself in the place of another is either an unconscious wish or guilt. In 'Group Psychology and the Analysis of the Ego', we see that identification with members of a group happens by putting the leader in the place of each of the member's ego ideal (Freud, 1921). I argue that we have in Freud a 'phenomenological gap' in what concerns the process of identification. There is little processual description nor a methodical study of the process of the way an object that is external gets to be taken 'on the inside'.

Ferenczi (1922b) introduces his particular conception of identification in a commentary on 'Freud's Group Psychology and the Analysis of the Ego' in 1922. Just like Freud, he has an understanding that the connection between group psychology and individual psychology is at the very foundation of psychoanalytic thought. Ferenczi assigns a precise libidinal place to identification:

> There is a libidinous process which runs parallel with this stage of ego-development and henceforward must be inserted as a special phase of development between narcissism and object-love (or, more correctly,

> between the still narcissistic oral and sadistic-anal stages of organization and true object-love). This process is identification.
>
> (Ferenczi, 1922b, p. 373)

This is a much more precise libidinal positioning of identification than in his earlier formulations (Ferenczi, 1912, p. 316), when the insistence was on introjection, described as a gradual extension of the original autoerotic interest to the external world. In other words, the ego takes in new objects, expanding the scope of its libido, and thus slowly enlarges itself.

In 1912, Ferenczi establishes the crucial distinction between *incorporation* and *introjection*, which I believe is at the heart of his theory of psychic fragments. Incorporation strikes us as a primarily oral act, where the object is as if 'swallowed whole' and not taken in gradually in its various aspects. By contrast:

> [in the introjection phase] objects are not really incorporated, as in the cannibalistic phase, but are 'incorporated' in an imaginary fashion, or, as we term it, introjected; that is to say, their qualities are annexed, attributed to the ego. The establishment of such an identification with an object (a person) is simultaneously the building of a bridge between the self and the outer world, and this connection subsequently permits a shifting of emphasis from the intransitive 'being' to the transitive 'having', i.e. a further development from identification to real object-love.
>
> (Ferenczi, 1922b, p. 374)

Introjection is thus an activity that pertains to Eros and to the very constitution of psychic life. We need to note that although at this point in time, 1912, Freud's discussion around the life drive had not yet taken place, we can understand introjection in relation to forces that prefigure the life drive, to activities of linking free psychic energy, and to assimilating more and more of what is outside the field of representation. Introjection is a particular way of taking in objects, where meaning is attributed at the same time of their 'handling'. Fantasy and sense-making accompany this process. As introjection happens, ever more complex 'psychic units' are created. In 1931, Alice Bálint, an important voice of the Budapest School of Psychoanalysis, reminds us that identification is central to the process of introjection, which she regards as a kind of 'mental digestion'. After her untimely death in 1939, a chapter from her Hungarian book was published in English in 1943. She writes: 'After this process of mental "digestion" has been successfully achieved, the object that had been so repellent only a short time before could now be held in the child's hands and felt as something friendly and familiar' (Bálint, 1943, p. 98). Psychic growth could thus be imagined as a 'concert of introjections' where several trails of fantasy and sense-making go on at the same time, enriching the psychic world and strengthening the ego.

What happens when this process of 'mental digestion' encounters difficulties? What are the vicissitudes of introjection? A first vicissitude emerges from the contrast proposed by Ferenczi between introjection and incorporation. If incorporation remains the main way of taking the world in, we could say we meet a psychic horizon of 'mental swallowing without digestion'. A second vicissitude is constituted by a relentless voracity of the introjective process. Ferenczi calls this excessive process 'neurotic introjection':

> the neurotic helps himself by taking into the ego as large as possible a part of the outer world, making it the object of unconscious phantasies. This is a kind of diluting process, by means of which he tries to mitigate the poignancy of free-floating, unsatisfied, and unsatisfiable, unconscious wish-impulses.
>
> (Ferenczi, 1909, p. 47)

What we are seeing here is an excess of phantasy, which produces the appearance of an overabundance of meaning, but which covers up a psychic reality where most of the energy is untied, free-floating. As Ferenczi (1909, p. 43) adds: 'The neurotic is constantly seeking for objects with whom he can identify himself, to whom he can transfer feelings, whom he can thus draw into his circle of interest, i.e., introject'.

As early as 1909, Ferenczi (pp. 48–49) articulates the ideas of 'projection' and 'primordial projection', which are the point of origin of all subsequent projections/introjections:

> We may suppose that to the new-born child everything perceived by the senses appears unitary, so to speak monistic. Only later does he learn to distinguish from his ego the malicious things, forming an outer world, that do not obey his will. That would be the first projection process, the primordial projection, and the later paranoiac probably makes use of the path thus traced out, in order to expel still more of his ego into the outer world.

> A part of the outer world, however, greater or less, is not so easily cast off from the ego, but continually obtrudes itself again on the latter, challenging it, so to speak; 'Fight with me or be my friend' (Wagner, Gotterdammerung, Act I). [...]
>
> The first 'object-love' and the first 'object-hate' are, so to speak, the primordial transferences, the roots of every future introjection.
>
> (Ferenczi, 1909, pp. 48–49)

As I have shown at length elsewhere (Soreanu, 2018a), Melanie Klein never entered into explicit dialogue with Ferenczi's notions of identification, projection and introjection. I argue that there is an important tension built into the Kleinian construction of 'projective identification', emerging from the very polarity of good object/bad object. The good/bad polarity functions as a proxy for a processual elucidation of psychic splitting, but it does not manage to do the phenomenological work that is needed for understanding what happens to the psyche at the time of splitting. There is thus no processual elucidation, no *quality* that can be added to describe the object, the internal phantasy of the object, or the effect the object has on the subject, which can diffuse the circular and perhaps morally coded relationship that the pair good/bad presuppose. I believe this moral duality and the circularity it inscribes (from good to bad and back again) gives a certain circularity to Klein's work, and to her conception of splitting in particular, where we move from projection to introjection and back again. There is thus a level of 'mundane' splitting assumed to be going on all the time in the psyche which does not dictate major metapsychological revisions or arrive at a metapsychology of fragmented psyches.

Psychic life is from the onset based on *qualities* and not on sheer polarities. We might be frustrated or satisfied, both by the object and in phantasy, but the question of remarkable significance is: in which particular way does frustration/satisfaction occur?

What we might miss if we remain faithful to the 'mundane' splitting that I discussed above is a more 'eventful' kind of splitting, resulting in de-libidinised (and re-libidinised) stable fragments of the psyche. In other words, we could say that fragments of the psyche become re-arranged in an enduring manner. There are very limited grounds in Melanie Klein's work to consider the tremendously difficult libidinal operation of projecting the bad or unwanted contents of the psyche. While this tremendous libidinal endeavour is attributed to very primitive states, we are left with the open question of whether, for such a successful and constant projection, a less primitive state of the ego is actually required, capable of channeling the libido in such a way that the unwanted contents can be discarded.

Yet another important difficulty with the Kleinian conception of splitting[2] rests in the fact that splitting functions in a silent or explicit duality with integration/cohesion. The psychoanalytic process itself is seen as aiming at achieving a better integration of the psyche. Working from the Ferenczian metapsychology of fragmented psyches, I argue that integration is not the polar opposite of splitting, nor is it the ultimate goal of analysis. Sometimes splitting is so profound, and results in such stable psychic fragments, that the psychoanalytic process is more accurately described as one of re-libidinisation of 'deadened' parts of the psyche.

In her 1946 piece 'Notes on Some Schizoid Mechanisms', Klein explains that, although we know little about the structure of the early ego, she is in agreement with Winnicott's emphasis on its unintegration. That is, the early ego lacks cohesion, or it alternates in its tendency towards integration and the opposite tendency of disintegration, a 'falling into bits' (Klein, 1946, p. 4). To deal with the anxiety arising from the operation of the death drive, the psyche creates an effect of fear of annihilation, which in its turn is reversed into fear of persecution. As Klein (1946, p. 4) stresses, the fear of the destructive impulse attaches itself at once to an object, which is experienced as a bad, overpowering object.

On the theme of splitting, she writes:

> The question arises whether some active splitting processes within the ego may not occur even at a very early stage. As we assume, the early ego splits the object and the relation to it in an active way, and this may imply some active splitting of the ego itself. In any case, the result of splitting is a dispersal of the destructive impulse which is felt as the source of danger. I suggest that the primary anxiety of being annihilated by a destructive force within, with the ego's specific response of falling to pieces or splitting itself, may be extremely important in all schizophrenic processes.
>
> (Klein, 1946, p. 5)

While Klein extensively detailed the first type of splitting – that done by the ego in relation to the object (what I referred to above as 'mundane' splitting, happening within the polarity of good object/bad object) – she leaves us to wonder what the more 'eventful' splitting of the ego into relatively stable fragments would look like. It is not sufficient to describe this type of splitting as 'psychotic' without explaining how it takes place and what movements of the libido it entails. We might want to ask: how do those fragments of the psyche that are not successfully projected, but 'stick' and arrange themselves in a stable form, appear to us?

It is worth mentioning that in her paper 'On Identification', Klein (1955) opts for a curious illustration of processes of splitting of the ego by analysing the novel *If I Were You*, written by French novelist Julian Green. In Green's story, a young clerk named Fabian Especel makes a pact with the Devil, which allows him to change himself into other people. Klein accompanies Fabian's journey through other bodies as he literally splits and projects his self into a new person/identity. Each of these transformations is accompanied by a new kind of disappointment and estrangement. Fabian both exits his body and remains in it.

I believe it is of great importance that Melanie Klein takes us to a work of fiction while working-through the ideas of identification, projection and splitting. Fabian is a product of fiction, and it is this fictionality that allows his massive projections onto others by literally inhabiting new bodies of choice. Perhaps in search of a more 'eventful' splitting of the ego (which would be encapsulated by Fabian's misrecognition of his old self when he enters the bodies of others, populated by their own traces and marks, and his sense of loss in relation to the part of the self that he had left in his old body), Klein curiously lands again in the realm of the splitting by the ego. Fabian's transformations remain metaphors of splitting, and no close equivalence of his body-travels can be established with actual patients or subjects. Thus, Fabian's journey is dreamed-up, phantasised; it is ultimately a series of 'mundane' projections. Klein writes:

> While it is important not to radicalize the distinction we proposed—between splitting by the ego, and splitting of the ego (to do so would mean to mis-recognize a point that Klein rightly directs us to in the above fragment, which is that any splitting by the ego brings into action a certain amount of splitting of the ego)—the question that remains unanswered relates to the psychic 'life' of the fragment that is the result of the splitting. What kind of metapsychology can allow us to talk

> effectively about the 'part of Fabian, lying dormant until the split-off aspects of his personality return'?
>
> (Klein, 1955, p. 166)

I would like to start answering this question by looking at one of Klein's late works, 'On the Development of Mental Functioning' (Klein, 1958), which brings a surprising metapsychological move. For the first time in her work, she introduces a kind of introjection where the 'terrifying figures' that used to be taken into the persecutory part of the superego are now relegated to a new unconscious place, a deep area of the unconscious, which remains untouched by regular developmental processes, and which has the capacity to overwhelm the ego. This move is intriguing, although it remains underspecified and enigmatic. It also comes in contrast to earlier views (see for instance the views expressed in the paper 'The Early Development of Conscience in the Child', written in 1933) where the normal early superego is precisely characterised by its extreme and terrifying nature.

We are thus talking about a novel kind of splitting, one that is stable and potentially irreversible: a splitting of the ego. The good object/bad object dyad and the moves of constant projection have only limited use for understanding this type of splitting. Melanie Klein never commented on this change of position, which I interpret here as radical. We are left to imagine the metapsychological consequences of her formulations, as well as possible forms of dialogue with other theorists (such as Ferenczi and his understanding of the 'identification with the aggressor', which I will discuss in the next section of this chapter).

In the paper 'On the Development of Mental Functioning', Klein (1958) discusses the two metapsychological principles that she inherited from Freud: his structural theory and his theory of the life drive and death drive. She states that the life and death drives are not general principles that function to support the biological life of the organism but rather a basis for love and hate, which are mental, not biological, phenomena.

In a section that partly addresses the 'phenomenological gap' of psychoanalysis on the problem of psychic splitting, she offers a description of how the superego is formed, through a fragmentation of the ego. She maintains that in this form of splitting both the life and the death drives find themselves predominantly in a state of fusion (Klein, 1958, p. 240).[3] It is here that Klein introduces a different kind of splitting and her 'terrifying figures' which in their destructiveness are not part of the superego. Instead, they exist in a separate area of the mind in the deep unconscious, split off both from the ego and the superego. They remain mostly unintegrated. A failure to keep these terrifying internal objects in a split-off area brings a state of overwhelming anxiety and endangers the equilibrium achieved among the other agencies of the psyche:

> When at the beginning of the twenties I embarked on the new venture of analysing by play technique children from their third year onwards, one of the unexpected phenomena I came across was a very early and savage super-ego. I also found that young children introject their parents—first of all the mother and her breast—in a phantastic way, and I was led to this conclusion by observing the terrifying character of some of their internalized objects. These extremely dangerous objects give rise, in early infancy, to conflict and anxiety within the ego; but under the stress of acute anxiety they, and other terrifying figures, are *split off in a manner different from that by which the super-ego is formed and are relegated to the deeper layers of the unconscious.*
>
> (Klein, 1958, pp. 240–241, my emphasis)

Klein's conclusion is that we are dealing with two kinds of splitting, one occurring in a state of fusion of the drives (which creates the superego); and one occurring in a state of diffusion of the drives (which creates the terrifying figures). While this second form of splitting remains enigmatic, it does launch a serious metapsychological challenge and it sketches possible paths of reflection on the problem of the nature and consequences of psychic splitting.

The difference in these two ways of splitting – and this may perhaps throw light on the many as yet obscure ways in which splitting processes take place – is that in the splitting-off of frightening figures diffusion seems to be in the ascendant; whereas superego formation is carried out with a predominance of fusion of the two instincts. Therefore, the superego is normally established in close relation with the ego and shares different aspects of the same good object. This makes it possible for the ego to integrate and accept the superego to a greater or lesser extent. In contrast, *the extremely bad figures are not accepted by the ego in this way and are constantly rejected by it* (Klein, 1958, p. 240, my emphasis).

I interpret Klein's surprising introduction of the 'terrifying figures' as a silent 'Ferenczian turn'. It is a matter of certainty that Klein was familiar with Ferenczi's formulation on the 'identification with the aggressor', which is one of the most phenomenologically thick accounts of psychic splitting that we possess in psychoanalysis to this day, and which we will turn to in the next section of this chapter. The identification with the aggressor stands at the very core of Ferenczi's conception of trauma.

Ferenczi shows how the fragile ego of the child is pulverised, atomised, and de-materialised in the moment of the trauma, only to take the shape afterwards, through a process of imitation, of the closest form that she encountered at the moment of the attack: the shape of the aggressor. I would say that this is the tragic side of the identification with the aggressor: it is, perhaps, best seen not as a mere introjection of the aggressor into a still-existing ego but as literally replicating the shape of the aggressor, at a time when the psyche has become no more than a cloud of disparate particles in search of a form. Let us remember Ferenczi's note in 'On Shock' (1932b, pp. 253–254), where he writes that in the hour of the attack the self is 'unfest, unsolid' and loses its form only to adopt an imposed form easily and without resistance, 'like a sack of flour'.

Having embarked on this plural Freudian, Kleinian, and Ferenczian journey, one possible conclusion is that there is psychic life beyond identification; or that a profound revision of our understanding of identification is called for. The psyche is capable of radical forms of plasticity and equally radical forms of splitting.

How to Make Sense of Fragments

Donna Haraway (2016, p. 10) writes: 'It matters what stories we tell to tell other stories with; it matters what concepts we think to think other concepts with'. It matters that in some of his notes of the *Clinical Diary* and in his 1924 book *Thalassa*, Ferenczi starts from the sea. He fantasises about life under water, inspired by the resilience of sea critters in times of catastrophe.

This brings a fresh direction to think with. In our times, voices of the 'blue humanities' start from the sea as a political act, placing cultural history in an oceanic rather than terrestrial context. Human civilisation and development have been situated mostly in pastoral fields, enclosed gardens or cities. What happens if we start from the sailor and swimmer, from the movement across oceans, and from estrangements at sea, rather than progressive settlements on land? One thing that happens is the perspective changes: it is no longer the gaze of the settler, encompassing the land from controlling heights, but the unsettled and uncertain view amid moving waters, ridden with doubts and the constant threat of dissolution. As Steve Mentz (2015) argues in *Shipwreck Modernity: Ecologies of Globalization, 1550–1719*, from an oceanic perspective, even the story of modernity is ultimately one of shipwrecks; it is a catastrophe-ridden epic where expansion happens in relation to sea crossings and to the many disasters waiting to happen. In our times traversed by migrant crises, and with boats capsizing while vulnerable humans try to get across borders and walls, it appears ever more important to start from the sea.

Jenny Willner (2023) followed the odd critters that populate Ferenczi's sea in *Thalassa* and showed their extraordinary importance in the attempt to make sense of psychic process and its extreme plasticity. Ferenczi (1924) establishes an analogy between sleep, dreams, sex life and the life of fantasy to look at a continuous regressive trend manifest in psychic life, which strives for the re-establishment of the intrauterine situation. But he also stays with the fish-becoming-amphibian, which is a reminder of the creative edge of catastrophe, of what the receding of the oceans can enable, in terms of creative adaptations and the formation of new organs and ultimately new forms of existence.

The spirit of this immersion in the sea is close to Haraway's 'sf', which stands for more than one thing. As she writes:

> The tentacular ones tangle me in sf. Their many appendages make string figures; they entwine me in the poiesis – the making – of speculative fabulation, science fiction, science fact, speculative feminism, *soin de ficelle*, so far. The tentacular ones make attachments and detachments; they make cuts and knots; they make a difference; they weave paths and consequences but not determinisms; they are both open and knotted in some ways and not others. sf is storytelling and fact telling; it is the patterning of possible worlds and possible times, material-semiotic worlds, gone, here, and yet to come. I work with string figures as a theoretical trope, a way to think-with a host of companions in sympoietic threading, felting, tangling, tracking, and sorting. I work with and in sf as material-semiotic composting, as theory in the mud, as muddle.
>
> (Haraway, 2016)

Both Haraway and Ferenczi share an interest in 'neural extravaganzas, fibrous entities, flagellated beings, myofibril braids, matted and felted microbial and fungal tangles, probing creepers, swelling roots, reaching and climbing tendrilled ones' (Haraway, 2016, p. 32).

What is important in Ferenczi's writing is that this keen interest in fish and amphibians does not amount to biologism or biological determinism. His 'bioanalysis' in *Thalassa* is an attempt to show the existence of a *psychic* sub-stratum manifest in all organic and inorganic matter. I believe his gesture of turning to sea critters is in resonance with contemporary feminist thinkers, who show us how to pay close attention to marine beings and to learn from their breathing techniques, their resilience, their modes of memory, their ways of splitting themselves into fragments and also of relating to one another. This is the case in Alexis Pauline Gumbs's (2020a, 2020b) book, *Undrowned: Black Feminist Lessons from Marine Mammals* and *Dub: Finding Ceremony.* As Gumbs (2020b, p. xiii) tells us, her project is 'an artefact and tool for breath retaining and interspecies ancestral listening'. And a few striking questions follow, all relating to interspecies imaginaries:

> what if you could breathe like whales who sing underwater and recycle air to sing again before coming up for air? What if you could breathe like coral from a multitude of simultaneous openings connected to one source built upon the bones of all your dead? What if you could breathe like cyanobacteria who made the sky into oxygen millions of years ago and sent their contemporaries to a world of sulphur deep under the ocean and ground?
>
> (Gumbs, 2020b, p. xiii)

All these questions invoke a radical plasticity, the ability to become-whale, and then become-coral, and then become-cyanobacteria. For Ferenczi, it is the scene of trauma that contains the possibility of such radical and surprising plasticity, as we will see in the following pages.

In *Thalassa*, Ferenczi invites us to his own psychoanalytic interspecies story of listening:

> Let me ask you to picture the surface of the earth as still entirely enveloped in water. All plant and animal life still pursues its existence in an environment of sea-water. Geologic and atmospheric conditions are such that portions of the ocean bed become raised above the surface of the

> water. The animals and plants thus set upon dry land must either succumb or else adapt themselves to a land and air existence; above all, they must become habituated to obtaining from the air, instead of from the water, the gases necessary to their existence – oxygen and carbon dioxide.
>
> (Ferenczi, 1924, p. 99)

In his poignant writing, Jakob Staberg (2023) reminded me of the atmosphere of a 'tactile eye' present in Ferenczi's work. This tactile mode of knowledge resonates with Haraway's post-humanist and feminist book *Staying with the Trouble* (2016, p. 30), where she talks about 'tentacular knowledge'. 'Tentacle' comes from the Latin *tentaculum,* which means 'feeler', and *tentare*, meaning 'to feel' and 'to try'. In making sense of Ferenczi's work, I encounter him as a 'tentacular' psychoanalyst and thinker: feeling, trying, experimenting, hesitating, advancing, retracting, revising; always relying on more than one sense or to a point of intersection (even confusion) between the senses, a synaesthesia. To follow the psychic life of fragments involves a descent into a depth, perhaps the depth of the sea or ocean. It also involves complex analogies between different kinds of catastrophes – ontogenetic, phylogenetic, geological, psychical.

What Can a Fragment Do?

In the *Clinical Diary*, Ferenczi (1932a, pp. 5–6) argues: 'under certain conditions, it can happen that the (organic, perhaps also the inorganic) substance recovers its psychic quality, not utilized since primordial times'; and

> [i]n moments of great need, when the psychic system proves to be incapable of an adequate response, or when these specific organs or functions (nervous and psychic) have been violently destroyed, then the primordial psychic powers are aroused, and it will be these forces that will seek to overcome disruption. In such moments, when the psychic system fails, the organism begins to think.
>
> (Ferenczi, 1932a, pp. 5–6)

What is surprising here is that the Freudian logic of hysterical conversion is turned on its head. In brief, for Freud, conversion is a scene where organs, limbs and nerves are transformed according to a psychic logic, which challenges strict anatomical laws. For Ferenczi, in contrast, there exists a 'language of organs' or a 'language of fragments', where various elements (tissue, limbs, cells, nerves) are arranged in meaningful relations. Anatomy is already impelled by psychic 'motives'.

In her book *Gut Feminism,* Elizabeth Wilson (2015) discusses the different perspectives on the relationship between the psyche and the soma in Freud's work and Ferenczi's work and some of the implications of this difference. In the Rat Man case history, Freud (1909, p. 157) argues that there is a 'leap from a mental process to a somatic innervation' that is characteristic of conversion hysteria, but he also claims that this leap 'can never be fully comprehensible to us'. In other words, there is a dissociation of somatic symptoms from anatomical constraint (Wilson, 2015). We are thus met with the image of a leap or a gap between the mental or the somatic, or a spatial divide between a psychic event and a bodily one. Conversion hysteria enigmatically bridges this gap, but we cannot account for *how* this bridging takes place. Furthermore, I believe that the Freudian text here puts psyche and soma in a hierarchical arrangement: the psyche *prevails* over anatomical laws and makes an inscription into the body, rearranging tissue, limbs, cells and nerves.

With Ferenczi, there is no leap, or gap, or enigmatic space between the psyche and the soma. Ferenczi brings a different solution, an escape from a 'flat biology', where the body is 'mere flesh'. Here, in this alternative 'n-dimensional biology', the biological stratum is also capable of different kinds of regressions, 'perversions, strangulations, condensations, displacements, which we usually attribute to the psychic stratum, or to non-biological systems' (Wilson, 2015). Ferenczi's work is thus surprisingly contemporary, in line with critiques of a reductionist, deterministic, flat and mechanistic understanding of matter.

In what follows, as we enter the scene of trauma, we encounter images of radical plasticity. The hysterical body is not a body possessed by fantasy, or by hallucinations, or by the psyche. It is a body that has gained 'semifluid' qualities, and where the tissue, limbs, cells and nerves speak the language of organs. Ferenczi's (1919) 'hysterical materialisations' involve a material transformation that does not cease to have meaning or to arrange elements in meaningful relations.

In a fascinating entry of the *Clinical Diary,* Ferenczi writes:

> if the psychically dormant substance is rigid, while the nervous and mental systems possess fluid adaptability, then the hysterically reacting body could be described as semifluid, that is to say, as a substance whose

> previous rigidity and uniformity have been partially redissolved again into a psychic state, capable of adapting. Such 'semisubstances' would then have the extraordinarily or wonderfully pleasing quality of being both body and mind simultaneously, that is, of expressing wishes, sensations of pleasure-unpleasure, or even complicated thoughts, through changes in their structure or function (the language or organs).
>
> (Ferenczi, 1932a, p. 7)

This gives an insight into the radical plasticity of the psycho-soma, where tissue, limbs, cells and nerves become capable of dream-like operations, of condensations and displacements.

While making sense of radical plasticity in the consulting room, the question 'what can an organ *do*?' (or 'what can a fragment *do*?') has been more useful to me than the questions 'what *is* an organ?' or 'what is an organ *for*?'. Paying attention to phenomena of hysterical materialisation means 'descending' into the body, listening to hearts, lungs and digestive tracts. Here, the hysterical lump in the throat is not just a hallucination, but it signals a new 'grammar' of organs. This grammar can animate the tissues of the throat, or the membranes of the heart, or the contents of the stomach. To put it in Jenny Willner's (2023, p. 115) terms, 'organs are not what they seem'. This is the terrain of a psychoanalysis of organs.

A psychoanalysis of organs means paying attention to the radical plasticity of organs, psychic fragments, blood vessels or nerve fibres that in certain circumstances are able to create new shapes or new configurations. New ad hoc organs are produced in the scene of trauma, and they become responsible for some of the organism's functions. 'Teleplasty' is a key term for Ferenczi's psychoanalysis of organs: it suggests a psychic act of moulding something at a distance or even an ex-corporation of organs, a kind of psychic ventriloquism. In some cases, the hallucination of breathing can maintain life, even where there is total somatic suffocation (Ferenczi, 1932a, p. 117). It is as if the subject generates ex-corporated lungs, which are the teleplastic double of the physical lungs. For the purposes of defence and survival, the subject can also generate 'receptacles, gripping tools, tools of aggression' (Ferenczi, 1932a) which will still fight for life, although the organism can find itself in a lifeless state or in deep coma. To further concretise this intriguing idea of teleplasty, Ferenczi evokes the case of 'R.N.' (Elizabeth Severn) who imagined an infinitely expandable bladder formed at the back of her head, where all her pain can accumulate (Ferenczi, 1932a,

p. 121). This pain-collecting bladder has a function in surviving the intensity of suffering in the scene of trauma. Ferenczi pays close attention in his clinical work to such odd organs, swelling up and disintegrating, in relation to some detail of the scene. Among these odd organs, the protective bladder has a special place, allowing some partial and hallucinatory integration in a psychic time where the danger of complete disintegration looms. We will turn to this in Chapter 3 of the book.

In *Thalassa*, Ferenczi (1924, p. 82) talks about an internal qualitative differentiation in the sphere of the libido, which can lead to an 'organ libido' and even an 'organ individuality'. As he writes:

> According to the 'theory of genitality', the cooperation of organs and of their component parts does not consist simply of the automatic adding together of useful workmen to give a sum total of performance. Each organ possesses a certain 'individuality'; in each and every organ there is repeated that conflict between ego- and libidinal interests which, too, we have encountered hitherto only in the analysis of *psychic individualities.*
>
> (1924)

Ferenczi differentiates between the 'altruistic' functioning of organs and autoerotic or self-gratifying processes in the tissues. Organs are thus capable of cooperation, but this is not a guaranteed outcome; it takes struggle and a complicated negotiation between opposing forces. At times, the cooperation collapses, and organs can work against one another.

In Chapter 3 of the book, we will follow Ferenczi in his construction of a new series of terms, which are both clinically and politically interesting, giving further grounding to the idea of 'altruistic' organs and fragments: cooperation, conciliation, endurance of suffering, selflessness, appeasement, adaptation to renunciation, self-denial, compromise. We will also look at how he experiments with a modification to the sphere of the dualism death drive/life drive. He renames them the 'drive of self-assertion' and the 'drive of conciliation' (Ferenczi, 1932a, p. 41). This 'selflessness' disposition or 'altruism' – including the 'selflessness' of organs – emerges in relation to the scene of trauma.

Another instance of radical plasticity I evoke here is that of a layering of organs: it appears that in the moment of trauma

> [n]ewly created organs in respect to their functions are only superposed upon the old without destroying them; even when the new functions make use of the material medium of the old, the latter organisation or function, although apparently given up, remains 'potential', 'biologically unconscious', and may again become active under certain circumstances.
>
> (Ferenczi, 1924, p. 93, fn)

This layering or superposition of organs means that any idea of evolution is questioned. The layered organs contain many times within themselves, many references to other moments, including other catastrophes. It is a curious concentricity of catastrophes, where forward movement or progress will almost certainly involve a level of denial of this multiplicity of temporal references.

What is the reason for all this recombinatory and plastic capacity of the psyche? Jenny Willner (2023) qualifies Ferenczi's *Thalassa* as a book of 'creatures that would have preferred not to conquer land'. This is a political image of self-limitation, of abstaining. The creatures that radically alter themselves to survive the catastrophe are not bound for glory. They have their own insurgent breathing techniques, their improbable forms of resilience, their modes of memory, their ways of splitting themselves into fragments, but also of cooperating with one another. The perspective in Ferenczi's writing turns away from a modernist narrative of progress: we do not meet the gaze of the settler, looking down upon the conquered land, but the unsettled and uncertain view of the sea creatures and their observer. They both seem to be located at sea, amid waves and overwhelming storms, facing the constant threat of sinking or dissolving. With Jenny Willner (2023, p. 119), we understand that in *Thalassa*, 'evolution is not a triumph, but a tragedy, the untold history of unmourned losses, a tale of survival that demands a new narrative'.

Revisiting the Scene of Trauma

Catastrophe and an Eventful Psychoanalysis

What does it mean to have survived a psychic catastrophe? What happens to the psyche at this time of catastrophe? With Sándor Ferenczi, we can imagine a catastrophe that is not a single, unitary event, but a *scene*, where several elements hold together in relation and interact – sometimes in a violent manner – and where certain structures and psychic positions are formed, and others destroyed. What kind of scene are we following here? How might we make sense of the different moves or psychic events that happen in this scene?

Catastrophe, event and trauma are at the core of Ferenczi's vocabulary. They are not identical or interchangeable terms, but together they constitute a way of talking about psychic processes that implies a series of important revisions to Freudian metapsychology. In what follows, with Ferenczi, we step into the domain of an *eventful psychoanalysis*. The images that predominate here are those of fractures, splits, atomisations, pulverisations, leakages, detritus, but also new formations, protective membranes, expansions, contagions, and inner growths. By reconsidering the scene of trauma, we take a further step towards making sense of the 'life' of the fragments that result from the splitting.

To the series catastrophe-event-trauma, we can add a fourth term: 'the shock of what is'. We can start with the voice of Cornelius Castoriadis (1989b): for him, 'the shock of what is' (*Anstoß*) is not a case of the environment causing a determinate outcome in the subject or in the living being. Instead, the kind of shock he has in mind 'sets in motion the formative (imaging/imagining, presenting and relating) capacities of the living being'. It is thus a sort of creative and consequential collision with the environment. This is already suggested in Fichte's original development of this idea. Literally, *Anstoß* is a 'stimulus' or a 'push'. For Castoriadis, just as for Ferenczi, the challenge is not to explain how the living being (or the subject) is determined by the environment but to explain how the living being's self-determination is *affected* by the environment. In other words, considering 'the shock of what is' means considering the fact that we have a relationship with the world that lies beyond our representations. It is, however, an encounter that sets in motion the process of representation that affects representations without determining them. Ultimately, this shock marks the self's capacity to be affected.

Set against the backdrop of this capacity of the self to be affected, the psychic catastrophe that I will capture in the following pages describes an *asymmetric encounter*, one between large and small, between powerful and vulnerable, between rigid and plastic. Indeed, we will see that Ferenczi's paradigm of relationality is an asymmetric one.

Asymmetry is written into what Ferenczi calls the 'confusion of tongues'. Trauma occurs in the form of a 'confusion of tongues' between the children and the adults. Children speak the 'language of tenderness', which is an experimental, playful and expansive register, through which more and more of the outside world is taken inside. Adults speak the 'language of passion', the register of adult sexuality, which has known repression and guilt. We can think of these two 'languages' as psychic registers that have their own modes of inscription. The meeting of the two languages causes children shock, a sense of intrusion, and an unbearable intensity. There is always some violence in the meeting of the two registers, as they do not just intersect or cross one another: instead, there is a clash, and the language of passion intrudes into the language of tenderness.

In describing the psychic effects of this encounter between the two registers – tenderness and passion – Ferenczi acts as a phenomenologist. In what follows, I revisit the scene of trauma in two ways. Firstly, with Ferenczi, I follow this phenomenological thread and discern how the fragile ego of the child is pulverised, atomised, de-materialised, only to afterwards take the shape, through a process of imitation, of the closest form that she encountered at the moment of the attack: the shape of the aggressor. I treat this as a new psychic process, a *psychic mimetism* that cannot be understood as a mere introjection of the aggressor into a still-existing ego. Instead, this psychic process has at its core a replication of the shape of the aggressor at a time when the psyche was almost entirely shapeless, or ego-less, and also very plastic, under the pressure of the traumatic attack. Let us remember here Ferenczi's note on the psyche being able to take on an imposed form easily and without resistance in the scene of trauma – the metaphor he uses to allow us to imagine this state is that of the psyche as 'a sack of flour' (Ferenczi, 1932b, pp. 253–254).

Secondly, I un-tie and re-tie this phenomenological thread by asking a series of questions about the different positions in the scene of trauma; about what is being included and what is being excluded from it; about the position from which the scene of trauma is assembled; about who is looking in and who is looking out, and who is doing the address and who is being addressed. It is important to make efforts to systematise Ferenczi's perspective, but it is equally meaningful to maintain some of the enigma of his 'confusion of tongues' which describes a state that is disorienting both to the subject and to any observer who meets traces of the scene of trauma. In the scene of trauma, the subject loses trust in their own senses and gives a big part of themselves to an other, to mould and use. A different other, who is watching over the repetition of the scene of trauma in another temporality, is also bound to feel disorientated as they percolate at the limit of what is knowable.

In engaging these questions, I draw on queer phenomenology and its vocabulary on disorientation. Disorientation is a form of non-normative postural subjectivation that encompasses non-mainstream inclinations, angles, and orientations. We can thus follow *oblique lines*, un-common *transversal trajectories*, and orientations that are *from below* or *from above*, which often happen in an encounter between small and large, between powerless and overpowering, between fixed and movable.

The confusion of tongues, as we will see below, is an *asymmetric encounter between two psychic registers*.

For Ferenczi, any traumatic event occurs in two moments and includes three presences. A first moment is when the language of passion intrudes into the language of tenderness (and this can take the form of an actual sexual assault or of a psychic transmission). The second moment is that of denial [*Verleugnung*], when a third adult called upon to recognise the intrusion fails to do so. It is only through the action of denial that an intrusive event becomes a trauma, bringing a near-death of the self, producing a gap in memory, and destroying the capacity of the subject to follow their own senses.

I include below a graphic representation of the grammar of the scene of trauma, referencing these three positions (Subject, Other of Aggression, and Other of Denial) and the two temporalities (the Time of Aggression and the Time of Denial).

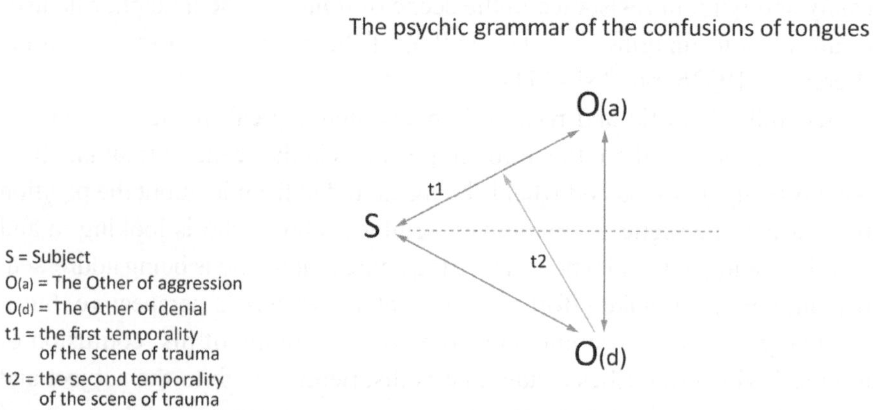

Figure 1.3 The Psychic Grammar of the Confusion of Tongues.

The 'confusion of tongues' is more than a narrow proposition for understanding sexual abuse and early trauma. It is a theory of the subject. The scene of the trauma that we will be disentangling over the next pages is also a scene of becoming-subject. For Ferenczi, no one can be 'outside' of the confusion of tongues. Existing purely in the register of tenderness is more of a clinical-theoretical fiction, which we need in order to better understand the encounter with the Other. Neither of the two registers can exist on its own; they are bound up together. In my interpretation, the register of passion is structurally prefigured in the register of tenderness. There is a structural *impossibility* of *not* having an encounter with the Other.

There are resonances here between Sándor Ferenczi and Jean Laplanche in terms of the importance given to the Other for the formation of subjectivity. For Laplanche, the subject is defined by the fact that she has an originary relationship with the enigma of the Other or with the enigmatic messages pertaining to adult sexuality. The originary mechanisms are not 'in person' but 'in otherness', and there is a constant reference to implantation (by the other) and to intromission (of something coming from the other) (Laplanche, 1999c, p. 257). What brings the two theorists together is a kind of 'clinical anthropology' that grounds their theories, establishing 'the child' and 'the adult' as different, not as developmental ages or as individual psyches but precisely as *psychic positions*. We are thus confronted with a universally asymmetrical situation.

The Scene of Trauma

Scenes can be regarded as a basic unit in the organisation of psychic matter. The Freudian *Nachträglichkeit*, translated by Jean Laplanche (1998) as 'afterwardsness', refers to a temporal logic that governs the psychic world, and where we have a system of 'scenes', a kind of psychic scenography emerging through the *interaction* effects between different moments in time (see also Baraitser, 2017; Birksted-Breen, 2003; Dahl, 2010; Faimberg, 2007; Fletcher, 2013). The traumatic consequences of the first scene are only released, in the form of a symptom, by the retrospective action of the second scene, which has the power to reactivate or revitalise the memory traces of the first scene. As Freud explains, the memory of the first scene persists, in a defensively isolated state, in a kind of limbo, or 'in storage'. The memory of the first scene is somewhat like a foreign body, composed via the excitation experienced at the time. The second scene reactivates it through associations and homologies. In other words, the initial memory of the first scene does not have any intrinsic power. It is only the interaction between the different temporalities that gives it its power, through processes of defence and repression.

John Fletcher (2013) points to Freud's insistence on the centrality of the first scene, traced back to an originary seduction scene. He refers to the other scenes as 'auxiliaries'. But the centrality of the first scene is only gained afterwards, through the occurrence of other subsequent scenes. Without the subsequent moments, we cannot speak of trauma in the first moment. This understanding supports the thesis of the sexual indifference or apathy of children. The memory traces of the first scene seem to be 'equal' for Freud. Any of them can be mobilised for a traumatic scenography of scenes.

In contrast, I would argue that the infantile ego is a *proto-ego*: a plastic, fragile, easy-to-overwhelm ego, unable to handle forms of stimulation that are too intense. Still, this proto-ego is neither apathetic nor indifferent; on the contrary, it is very sensitive to the moments when adults cease to address it in what Ferenczi referred to as 'the language of tenderness' and start to address it in the incomprehensible 'language of passion'. Not all memories thus have the potential of subsequent contribution to the complicated composition of scenes and temporalities that can constitute a 'trauma'. It is only the marks resulting from the clash between the language of passion and the language of tenderness that produce the 'pool' of memories of the scene of trauma.

For Ferenczi, language imitates the body and body parts in a complicated manner. This means that associations have a *necessary* aspect to them, and thus they also need to be very *precise*. Marion Oliner (2013) has recently drawn to our attention that although there is a growing body of work in psychoanalytic theory on the irrepresentable, the non-represented, or the non-represented mental states, we are still confronted with an unsettling clinical-empirical puzzle in the fact that there is often a very striking *accuracy* in the enactments and actualisations of the traumatic events, even when the memory of them remains inaccessible to consciousness. This is to say that the psycho-soma is able to re-stage the traumatic events with a great level of precision. This precision and minuteness of detail leads us to believe that it is not that these marks were not presented in any way to the psyche or that they belong to the realm of the irrepresentable. Oliner (2013) uses 'non-represented' in inverted commas, drawing our attention to the overuse of this term to cover situations where what is actually missing are the associations between different modes of representation (or, we would say, between different modes of presentation in the psyche). We have seen above that the memory of the id and the memory of the ego have different manners of retaining a mark. What we often regard as 'non-represented' actually refers to marks that were retained only in the memory of the id, as affects or life and death trends, and were not tied with marks of the memory of the ego.

I understand this as a significant challenge to the thesis of the infantile sexual indifference. Aspects of the scene of trauma linger on. The scar-tissue of memory is formed in relation to the particular way in which the proto-ego was wounded.

The differential of Ferenczi's understanding of the scene of trauma lies in structuring it around a third presence, which 'locks-in' the trauma via denial (or misrecognition of the nature or of magnitude of the child's experience, whose world was broken by the intrusion of the language of passion of the adult). When, in a clinical setting, different registers of memory become linked to one another, and the memory of the id becomes connected in stronger ways to the memory of the ego, what we achieve are *effects of authenticity*. Originally, the trauma brought the splitting of the ego, producing *effects of inauthenticity*. It is crucial to mark that the memory of the id is capable of some form of inscription. This means that, both in 'locking-in' the trauma and in its subsequent unpacking and working-through, the memory of the id has a leading role. The reliving of a different moment in time and the recuperation of the split-off parts of the ego unfold *in the spirit of the marks inscribed via the memory of the id.*

Traumatic Imitation

In what follows, I argue that Ferenczi's formulation on the 'identification with the aggressor' is one of the most phenomenologically thick accounts of psychic splitting that we possess in psychoanalysis to this day. The identification with the aggressor stands at the very core of Ferenczi's conception of trauma, as many contemporary authors have shown (Frankel, 1998;

2015; Lénárd & Tényi, 2003). The identification that Ferenczi talks about is a tragic one: it contains a primary element of *imitation* of form and an *introjection of guilt feelings*. This introjection of the guilt feelings, however 'dark' in itself, allows the child to continue living after having gone through an overwhelming and potentially deadly experience. In a note in his *Clinical Diary*, in an entry of 10 May 1932, the kind of splitting that Ferenczi (1932a, p. 103) describes appears to be qualified: it is not a split between good and bad, but instead between reason and emotion. The two faculties become separated from one another and gain quasi-autonomous functioning. Both become hyper-faculties – enhanced but also split.

Unlike Anna Freud's (1936) idea of the 'identification with the aggressor', Ferenczi's does not wish to capture a kind of ego defence, where an aggressor is taken as the object of identification by a (quite mature) ego. Instead, what Ferenczi means by his 'identification with the aggressor' refers to a much more complicated and primary process. Here, the notions of de-materialisation and traumatic imitation are crucial: he uses terms such as pulverisation (*Pulverisierung*) and atomisation (*Atomisierung*). Ferenczi does not use these terms as metaphors. Instead, he has in mind particular moments in the traumatic scene, when the ego is literally pulverised into bits, and when it loses whatever stable shape it had before.

The process of pulverisation assumes the existence of a kind of 'proto-ego'. There is always some form that can be shattered through traumatic shock or the confusion of tongues, even for an ego that is not very developed. Pulverisation is accompanied by both positive and negative hallucinations. Through the positive hallucinations, the subject reverts to the previous state of tenderness that preceded the trauma, with its clash between the register of tenderness and the register of passion. It is as if a voice was uttering, 'I wish to exist in a time *before* this happened to me'. Through the negative hallucinations, the subject creates a psychic position grounded in asserting, 'This is not happening to me'. We can see that this position produces a fundamental alteration of the reality principle: the subject has in their repertoire the denial of overwhelming and unpleasant feelings, often through a combination of negative and positive hallucinations.

In a fragment from 1930 titled 'Each Adaptation is Preceded by an Inhibited Attempt at Splitting', Ferenczi (1930b) prefigures the possibility of psychic reconstruction out of the fragments of the traumatic attack. He notes that even fragments that are apparently shapeless, that bear no articulation with the ego, and that appear to us as mere 'psychic energies' (marking a sort of reversibility of the formation of the ego from instinctual forces, a re-falling into the realm of the drives) can serve as a ground for psychic reconstruction:

> In the extreme case when all the reserve forces have been mobilized but have proved impotent in the face of the overpowering attack, it comes to an extreme fragmentation which could be called dematerialization. Observation of patients, who fly from their own sufferings and have become hypersensitive to all kinds of extraneous suffering, also coming from a great distance, still leave the question open whether even these extreme, quasi-pulverized, elements which have been reduced to mere psychic energies do not also contain tendencies for reconstruction of the ego.
>
> (Ferenczi, 1930b, p. 220)

Respecting a psychic rule where any form is better than no form, a part of the psyche pulverised by the power of the traumatic attack borrows the shape of that which is closer: the shape of the aggressor. This is a phenomenon of traumatic imitation that brings into being one of the deadliest fragments of the psyche: a fragment that performs a direct mimicry of the manner or the psychic ways of the aggressor. From a kind of 'cloud of particles', the psyche stabilises into the form of the aggressor. This insight is important for understanding how intergenerational transmission of trauma takes place: it will undoubtedly involve phenomena of traumatic imitation, by which a traumatic residue will *intrude* in the psyche, causing first a dematerialisation and afterwards a re-materialisation that observes the form of the aggressor.

Guilt is therefore the enigmatic and violent transmission that comes from the Other. This is because in the clash between the language of passion and the language of tenderness, the language of passion – that of the adult – is structured precisely around guilt and repression. Here, we would have to distinguish traumatic guilt from neurotic guilt. Traumatic guilt is a catastrophic and non-neurotic kind of guilt: it is sudden, and it propels the subject into a state of traumatic confusion after having received this 'alien transplant'.

There is one section of Ferenczi's 1933 text on the 'confusion of tongues' that I believe produces significant insights for clinicians: I have experienced how powerful it is to teach around it or unpack it in a clinical group.

I think this is because Ferenczi gives a precise phenomenological insight about how a fragment of the psyche comes into being:

> These children feel physically and morally helpless, their personalities are not sufficiently consolidated in order to be able to protest, even if only in thought, for the overpowering force and authority of the adult makes them dumb and can rob them of their senses. *The same anxiety, however, if it reaches a certain maximum, compels them to subordinate themselves like automata to the will of the aggressor, to divine each one of his desires and to gratify these; completely oblivious of themselves they identify themselves with the aggressor.* [...]
>
> The most important change, produced in the mind of the child by the anxiety-fear-ridden identification with the adult partner, is *the introjection of the guilt feelings of the adult* which makes hitherto harmless play appear as a punishable offence.
>
> (Ferenczi, 1933, p. 162)

What Ferenczi describes here is how the aggressor ceases to be a part of external reality (extrapsychic) and instead becomes intrapsychic. What he calls 'identification with the aggressor' or 'introjection of the aggressor' actually presents itself as an 'incorporation of the aggressor'. The psyche of the victim 'swallows' the aggressor whole as if in a single psychic act. This 'swallowing up' is centred on the guilt feelings, which represent one of the least 'metabolisable' psychic facts of the scene. If we refer to the phenomenon of traumatic imitation, we can say that non-neurotic guilt functions as the necessary core of the imitation. We are dealing with a new psychic organisation, structured around guilt.

The suddenness of this incorporation creates a trance-like state which is dominated by 'positive or negative hallucinations' (1933). As reality has become too terrifying, the hallucinations serve a precise function. The positive hallucinations restore the situation of tenderness, or the situation before the intrusion of the language of passion into the language of tenderness. In other words, the child recreates in fantasy the pre-traumatic state, which has been lost. The negative hallucinations manifest themselves as an overwhelming feeling of 'being bad', because the 'wrongness' of the traumatic scene has been incorporated and curved inwards. All aggression is now masochistically directed towards the inside. Frankel (2015) has discussed the facets of this traumatic feeling of 'badness' in the contemporary clinic.

This 'badness' results from the child taking upon himself the badness that resides in his objects. We could say that this 'badness' is a negative hallucination of a very particular sort, which takes a part of the self as the object. The ego punishes the subject through a kind of 'strike', through hypersensitivity and lack of energy. As Ferenczi (1932a, p. 188) puts it, '[c]ertain observations suggest that an oppressive sense of guilt can occur even when one has not transgressed against oneself at all'.

The result of this catastrophic incorporation is that the child enters a state of traumatic confusion where the 'confidence in the testimony of his own senses is broken' (Ferenczi, 1933, p. 162). In other words, the child now confuses inner and outer reality and is dominated by an omnipotence of thoughts where it becomes impossible to distinguish what is imagined from what is real. This is the result of 'knowing terrible things' (Bragin, 2007; Benjamin, 2018).

There are important political implications deriving from the existence of such a psychic position. Bragin (2007) argues that victims of torture experience the fear that some hidden and terrible badness resides in them. They start to believe that their own childhood fantasies of harm are congruent, deciphered, and enacted by the perpetrator, who can somehow respond to their own pre-existing internal choreography of destructiveness. Thus, they start to feel that they resemble their torturer in their own familiarity with the 'terrible things'. These 'terrible things' and the hallucinations that surround them bind the victim and the perpetrator together, because there emerges a sense of sharedness in something that others are ignorant of. The originary traumatic confusion thus creates an omnipotent belief in one's own badness that allows further forms of abuse and exploitation to take place. This form of 'being bad' is incompatible with feelings of self-esteem or worth.

The psychic fragment that results from the incorporation of the guilt feelings of the aggressor is directly implicated in social compliance and submission. Any demand of 'blind' compliance, which does not entail a deliberative process, will appeal to the 'mechanical, obedient automaton' that the subject was reduced to in the scene of the trauma.

The phenomenon of hyper-attunement with the feelings and intentions of the aggressor has a role in maintaining structures of domination. At the time of the attack, the child forms the fantasy that they sense the aggressor needs from them, which increases the chances of surviving the terrifying situation. On the one hand, this means developing hyper-sensitivities and hyper-intuitions. On the other hand, it means failing to perceive certain aspects of reality, which would counter the traumatic 'script' that was implanted in the child or that would threaten the hyper-attuned traumatic adaptation. We could thus say that while certain aspects of reality are hyper-perceived, others are dissociated from. Any political system of domination will demand from its subjects similar kinds of traumatic 'selectiveness' that result in perfect mental and behavioural compliance. The atrocities and murders of the regime are to be erased from memory, while the political rituals that maintain and celebrate the regime are to be diligently observed.

A new important series of terms emerges in the *Clinical Diary:* guilt, implantation of an alien will, alien transmission, alien transplant. Guilt is the object of the enigmatic and violent transmission that comes from the Other.

Orientations, Inclinations and the Scene of Trauma

In the account of the scene of trauma I have given so far, there are many *oblique lines*, un-common *transversal trajectories*, orientations that are *from below* or *from above*, which often happen in an encounter between small and large, between powerless and overpowering, between fixed and movable.

Phenomenology and psychoanalysis share an interest in how objects and bodies acquire orientations or inclinations to one another, in the way they come to 'point' to each other. Bodies acquire such orientations or inclinations through reiterative action or repetition of certain gestures. These repetitions have particular 'objects' in view, but these are only sometimes material or physical objects (the psychoanalytic couch, the chair, the consulting room door); other times they are psychic, or fantasy objects that bear an investment or identification (the psychoanalytic frame, the psychoanalyst's position, the boundaries of the psychoanalytic process). I draw on phenomenological ideas of 'orientation' and 'inclination', as they can help us in capturing the tension between the fugitive and the reiterative nature of action, and in approaching the grammar of the scene of trauma. Sara Ahmed (2006) and Adriana Cavarero (2016) are important partners of dialogue here, as they both use geometrical/spatialised metaphors to rethink subjectivity and ethics (see also Dahms, 2023). Their explorations of subjectivity through postural (inclined) and spatial (oriented) lines and relations mean that we can enter the grammar of the scene of trauma. This line of theorising also brings an ethical bind. According to Ahmed (2006, p. 95), 'to think with orientations is to think of how we are involved in worlds; it is to write from our involvement'.

It would be a dangerous illusion to think that orientations and inclinations are always readily visible or easy to capture. A psychoanalytic phenomenology insists on the force of phantasy in organising the geometric metaphors that Ahmed and Cavarero speak about. There is always something *behind* or *beneath* the field of perception that we need to pay attention to. What falls behind or beneath is not neutral, but it often has to do with racialisation and the production of whiteness. As Sara Ahmed (2006, p. 133) writes: '[t]he institutionalization of whiteness involves work: the institution comes to have a body as an effect of this work'. Here, Frantz Fanon's voice is important, pointing to the orientations *beneath* other corporeal orientations, which he calls 'historical-racial schema':

> Below the corporeal schema I had sketched out a historic-racial schema. The elements that I used had been provided for me not by 'residual sensations and perceptions primarily of a tactile, vestibular, kinaesthetic, and visual character', but by the other, the white man, who had woven me out of a thousand details, anecdotes, stories.
>
> (Fanon, 1986, p. 17)

What we take from this is that the racial and historical dimensions are *beneath* and *below* the surface of the body. What we also take from this is that in any analytical exploration of how to approach the scene of trauma, we need to observe the constant orientation of 'weaving out' Black and marginal subjects of details, anecdotes and stories.[4]

Even while considering that the scene of trauma is structured and has a grammar, it is important to register moments of disorientation with instances when what is straight or aligned becomes *oblique* or *diagonal* or gains a new angle. What is assumed here is a conflicted subject who becomes disorientated by their own conflict while also disorienting their audience or observer. I am drawing on multiple insights in queer phenomenology, which offers a whole vocabulary around disorientation and understands it as a form of non-normative postural subjectivation. As Lauren Berlant and Michael Warner (2005, p. 198) write, the 'queer world is a space of entrances, exits, unsystematized lines of acquaintance, projecting horizons, typifying examples, alternate routes, blockages, incommensurate geographies' (2005, p. 198). Sara Ahmed talks about seeing the world 'slantwise' (2006, p. 107), which means that objects and bodies that are not usually woven into the story get to come into view. Ultimately it is important to note, in resonance with Ahmed, that disorientation has an uneven distribution in the world: some bodies, those of minorities, Black people, women, trans subjects, get to be more often disorientated.

What are the implications of this attempt to follow the disorientations? Here we return to Adriana Cavarero's notion of 'inclinations' which unpacks subjectivity in postural and relational terms. With her book *Inclinations: A Critique of Rectitude*, we become aware of the gestures, alignments and disalignments of all those in history who, through their work of care, are more visibly inclined towards others. What results is a hidden geometry of postural care. Cavarero looks at how Western philosophy has produced a core image of a subject that is vertical, straight and self-balanced, and who holds himself upright in relation to every other subject: the autonomous 'I'. This 'formal uprightness' (Cavarero, 2014) is also a paradigm of relationality: it configures the way in which care, social roles, norms, deviance, bodies will be grasped. What is here woven out of the story is the 'inclined I', the subject who is not straight or vertical but oblique or tilted. This is the obliqueness of care and preoccupation with others. Cavarero refers to a quality of this inclination that is 'leaning toward the outside' (2014). It is this quality of subjectivity that interests us as well, approaching both the scene of trauma and the way the scene of trauma is written/imagined by various psychoanalytic authors (Freud, Ferenczi, Laplanche). What does it mean to start imagining a subject position that is articulated around the act of leaning *toward the outside*?

The Diagonal Position

I free associate here with a scene of psychoanalytic obliqueness. It is a scene around the 1960s in Brazil, when psychoanalyst Katrin Kemper (later to become the founder of the psychoanalytic society Círculo Psicanalítico do Rio de Janeiro) proposed two interrelated interventions into the psychoanalytic *dispositif*. The first is the 'mutative-alluded interpretation' [*interpretação mutativa aludida*], which pays attention to the 'atmosphere' of the communicative act and to nonverbal communication. What matters is *how* things are being uttered, in terms of their 'atmospheric transmissions', in terms of rhythm, but also in terms of the interruptions and incomplete sentences of the analyst herself, of her isolated sounds, gestures or facial postures (Kemper, 1962). This intervention is paired up with another one, which 'tilts' the 'classical position' of the analyst in her analytic chair that dictates the analyst should sit fully behind the patient/couch. Kemper proposes exploring a revision to this position, and she refers to it as the 'diagonal position', which would allow the patient to develop a fantasy of being at least partially watched or visible and also having, if needed, some perception of the analyst's gaze. As she writes:

> The possibility of perception of silent transmissions is, in my view, limited by the classical position of the analyst. The analyst's 'diagonal position', that is, the fact that he is seated behind and right beside the patient, allows better than the classic position the observation of mute communications expressed by mimic, gestures and everything that is expressed in an obvious way by way of movement. I think that the 'diagonal position' allows the patient, to perceive and look at the analyst as much as he needs do; likewise, it enables the analyst to better perceive silent transmissions. See Th. Benedek's conception (sitting behind the patient may correspond to a running away by the analyst).
>
> (Kemper, 1962)[5]

In what follows, I trace the way Sándor Ferenczi's writings on the scene of trauma can be read, while I pay attention to orientations, inclinations, obliqueness and diagonals.

The Child in the Scene of Trauma: A New Optics

What are the positions in the scene of trauma? What is excluded from it? And from which perspective is it unfolding? Who is looking in? Who is looking out? Who is doing the address? Who is being addressed? The ideas of *orientation* and *inclination* discussed thus far are important for engaging these questions.

As I showed above, what brings theorists such as Laplanche and Ferenczi together is the kind of 'clinical anthropology' that grounds their theories, which establishes 'the child' and 'the adult' as different, not as developmental ages or as individual psyches, but precisely as *psychic positions*. With this, we are in a universally asymmetrical situation.

What are the inclusions and exclusions in terms of the grammar that is being proposed? And what kind of 'optics' of the trauma scene do the two authors (Ferenczi and Laplanche) bring? From whose perspective is the trauma scene written? What is particular to the Ferenczian scenography of the psyche? And what kind of orientations and inclinations bind the elements of the scene together? The first thing to note is that for Ferenczi, *the child is included in the trauma scene. The child is not looking from the outside or looking in on a scene in which the adults are acting.* In Laplanche, the psychic act belongs to the adults, as they are (unconsciously) *addressing* the child via their actions/interactions/intercourse. As Laplanche (1997, p. 661) points out: 'showing sexual intercourse is never simply an objective fact, and that even the letting-see on the part of the parents is always in a sense a making-see, an exhibition' [...] 'a message, a giving-to-see or a giving-to-hear'.

The *figure of the child* stands at the centre of Ferenczi's theory of trauma and scenography of trauma. *The scene is organised from the perspective of the child.* The psychic position of the child acts and responds to the aggression and denial of the Other: it splits itself into fragments, it even de-materialises itself, it traumatically imitates the aggressor's shape, but it also creates a new psychic organisation out of the fragments.

It is not surprising that Ferenczi was able to experiment with these 'optics' that include the child. For him, the child is a figure that is meaningful – philosophically, sociologically and clinically. It would perhaps be more accurate to speak of Ferenczi's 'children', as there are different hypostases of the child that populate his world. Firstly, there is the actual child, the one who suffers the trauma and enters the triangle of the confusion of tongues. This child makes herself present – in the consulting room, in the analysis of the adult (Ferenczi, 1931a), in the process of repeating the infantile trauma, in the presence of the analyst. Secondly, there is the 'wise baby' – a psychoanalytic construction that has come to stand for the process of splitting and for the radical separation between reason and emotion. Thirdly, there is Orpha – a fragment of the psyche, formed in the process of splitting, which also acquires qualities of a true novel psychic agency, constituting one of Ferenczi's most important theoretical inventions. (Chapter 3 of this book is dedicated to Orpha.) Fourthly, there is *homo infans*, a philosophical construction at the centre of Ferenczi's idea of the emancipated subject. *Homo infans* is the post-traumatic subject who has touched the wounds and scars of childhood and is unafraid of the experience of being in fragments and living by the fragments, without any total integration into a single coherent identity.

The fact that the scene of trauma is written from the perspective of the child creates a series of orientations and oblique lines. As Ferenczi notes, what is incessantly replayed in the scene of trauma is the encounter between an 'over-great (fat) aggressor' and 'a much smaller, weaker person, oppressed and dominated by the aggressor' (Ferenczi, 1930c, p. 228). How can we further imagine this situation of asymmetry? I have been thinking of it as an *oblique line pointing upwards*.

To an extent – by virtue of its organisation across three presences (Subject, Other of Aggression and Other of Denial) and two distinct temporalities (the Time of Aggression and the Time of Denial) – the scene of trauma in Ferenczi is much more structured than it is in Freud and in Laplanche. In Laplanche, if we consider the sentence/scene 'father seduces daughter', the subject can take any place in the scene: they can be 'father' or 'seduces' or 'daughter'. For Ferenczi, the circulation between the positions depends on the depth and extent of psychic fragmentation and on the fate of the identification with the aggressor in the history of the subject. While it is the scene itself that is introjected, and while there will always be some phantasmatic circulation between the three positions, not all three of them will be equally available to the subject.

Ferenczi writes his theory from the inside out, from within the scene of trauma. In terms of orientation, he experiments with the oblique line pointing upwards. This line is psychically drawn by a small, vulnerable, and plastic subject who is confronting an Other who is more powerful, authoritative, and fixed than themselves.

The Position of the Analyst: A New Optics

The analyst's position has a fundamental relationship to the act of denial. We can say that it is structured in relation to denial. The analysis allows a reliving of the original conflict between the ego and the environment and the painful solutions the subject found for this conflict. The orientation of this reliving is to search for fresh solutions. This revision of the trauma scene needs to take place in 'new conditions' which can lead to a new psychic resolution for the patient and a re-arrangement of the psychic fragments. The new conditions are predicated on the analyst's different relationship to denial and recognition. Ferenczi argues that

> [t]he most essential aspect of the altered repetition [of the scene of trauma] is the relinquishing of [the analyst's] own's rigid authority and the hostility hidden in it. The relief that is obtained thereby is then not transient and the convictions derived in this way are also more deeply rooted.
>
> (Ferenczi, 1932a, p. 108)

In other words, the analyst will experiment with not taking a position of authority and not demanding submission. Their orientation in the scene will not be one of looking from above, but from beside or from below. Their position will be *different* to the situation in childhood, which was one of suggestion and of the emergence of infantile obedience in the form of a psychic scene played and replayed between a small vulnerable being and a big overpowering one.

In the *Clinical Diary*, Ferenczi refers to mutuality as an 'antidote' to the hypnotic lies in childhood. The analyst's intervention will have an effect of *demechanisation* or *dehypnotising*. This implies a (partial) reversibility of psychic processes of fragmentation. The psychic state of functioning as an 'automaton' – which was produced in the process of identifying with the aggressor – is at least in part reversible. The 'traumatophilic' nature of the analytic space that Ferenczi invites us to imagine means that while getting close to wounds, scars and scar-tissues, the analysis makes possible 'the recognition and assertion of one own's self as a genuinely existing, a valuable entity of a given size, shape, and significance' (Ferenczi, 1932a, p. 129).

I would like to qualify the recognition that is at play here. It is not the kind of recognition that conditions the very existence of the subject and that gets us bound up in the Master-Slave dialectic. Denial is prior to recognition. Recognition here is not an extra-social act or one that precedes the relationship. Recognition is a secondary act which precipitates a re-arrangement of the fragments. I call this particular kind of analytic act *reconstructive recognition*. This reconstructive recognition is not organised in relation to some historical or biographical 'truth', or to the way things 'really were' in the scene of trauma, but in relation to the magnitude of suffering of the subject. It responds to traces of catastrophic suffering while not denying their catastrophic quality. The analyst's position in relation to the magnitude of suffering makes a new inscription following the grammar: *where denial was, recognition shall be.* I call this the first grammar of the analytic act of recognition.

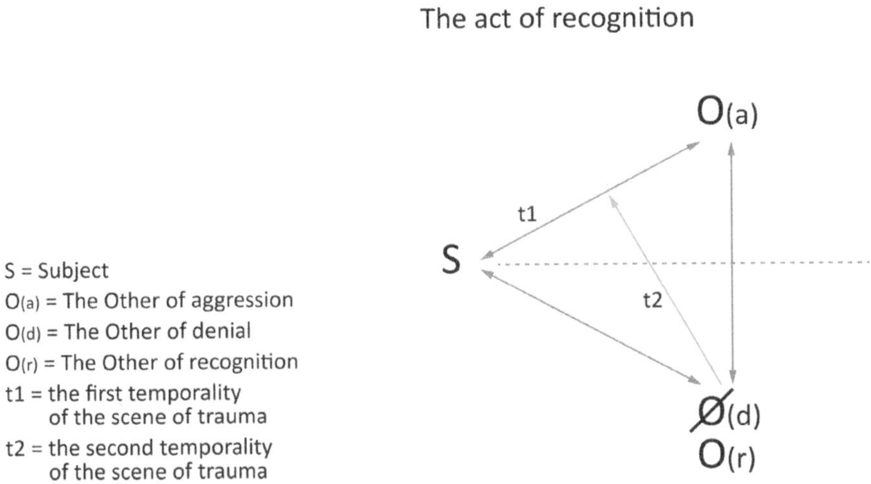

Figure 1.4 The First Grammar of the Analytic Act of Recognition.

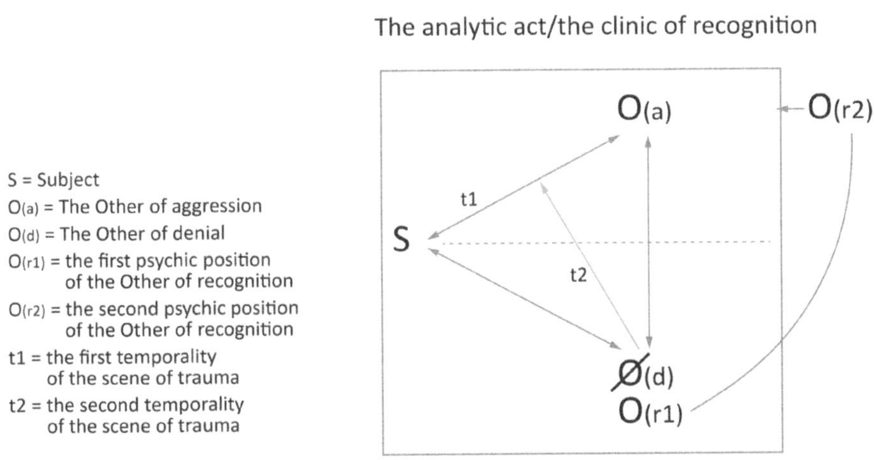

Figure 1.5 The Second Grammar of the Analytic Act of Recognition.

What is then the second grammar of the analytic act of recognition? Apart from the magnitude of suffering, the analyst recognises the very existence of a confusion of tongues, of a scene of trauma which contains three positions: victim, aggressor and agent of denial. The confusion of tongues is a grammatical, structuring, psychic fact which creates a singular psychic organisation. The analyst does thus not expect the subject to be always fixated on and identified with the position of 'victim' but knows that their psychic repertoire contains the positions of 'aggressor' and 'agent of denial' as well. One understanding of psychic plasticity is referring precisely to the ability to circulate between these positions. This constitutes perhaps the single type of *knowledge* that the analyst has in addition to the patient: it is a kind of grammatical knowledge, a consciousness of the importance of 'scenes', and a sensibility geared to 'scenes' and their ramifications in terms of psychic fragmentation and psychic suffering. The two types of analytic recognition work together and complement each other, in such a way that the analyst is *never only within* the scene of trauma, identified with one or the other of its positions; and *never only outside* the scene of trauma, looking in from above, as a distant observer. This *neither-only-within-nor-only-without* or *both-within-and-without* creates its own obliqueness. It avoids fixing one in the position of master, and another in the position of slave, and instead it grapples with the challenges that come from occupying more than one position and being more than one to the other.

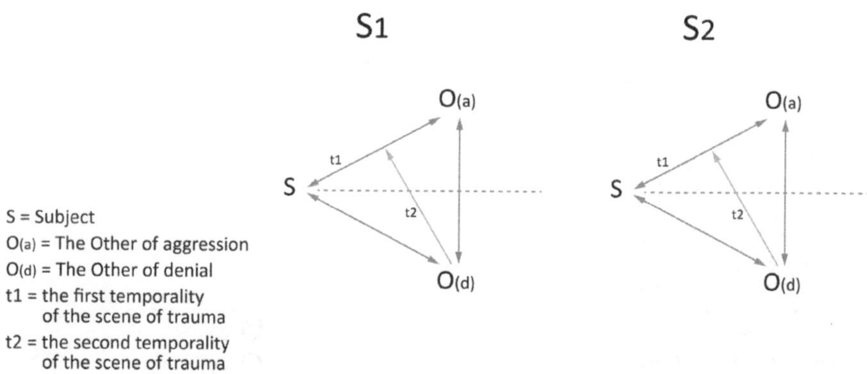

Figure 1.6 An Interpretation of the 'Dialogue of Unconsciouses' in Sándor Ferenczi.

It is essential to add a further note to the observation on the grammatical knowledge of the analyst and their sensibility geared to scenes. The analyst also knows there are *two* subjects in the consulting room, and neither of them can stand 'outside' the confusion of tongues. In other words, the analyst knows that they also subject to moving between the positions of victim, aggressor and agent of denial. In the *Clinical Diary*, Ferenczi approaches the analytic relationship as a system co-constructed by two parties, and he speaks of a 'dialogue of unconsciouses' (Ferenczi, 1932a, p. 84). Transference and countertransference also make up a system, and we cannot make sense of one without the other.

Ultimately, the analysis is work with fragments. There are moments of re-arrangement of fragments or even of re-fashioning a new (partial) unit from debris and shattered pieces. There are moments of attempting to link up the fragments, so that they don't exist in complete isolation from one another. I read all these acts as *oblique* acts: the analyst is never above this scene of fragments, having mastery over the scene, but somehow beside it, lateral to it, in a state of *passiblity* (Scarfone, 2019; Baraitser, 2023) or *oblique stillness* – sometimes pointing away from the scene and sometimes pointing to the scene. The analyst balances between changing positions and being still – or bearing, at least for a while, the position that the other is putting (or pushing) them into.

The implication of the existence of a psychic orientation of oblique stillness is that we can come to imagine, clinically and politically, a form of *resistance to the identification with the aggressor* and all the psychic violence that comes with it (psychic de-materialisation, imitation of the shape of the aggressor, fixation in the position of the aggressor). In his talk at the International Sándor Ferenczi Conference in São Paulo in June 2024, psychoanalyst Endre Koritar spoke about the hypnotic influence of political leaders in our times and asked important questions about the possibilities of *resistance* to the identification with the aggressor. Ferenczi's (1932a) note on 'the dialogue of unconsciouses' is relevant here, marking the fact that there are always at least two subjects in a scene, two unconsciouses in entanglement. As we saw above, each of the subjects in their turn has internalised the grammar of the scene of trauma, so each of them has three distinct positions available to them. Thus, any impasse or creative outcome between the two subjects can be imagined as a series of (oblique) lines that pass between the different psychic positions that each of the subjects has available (victim, aggressor, and agent of denial). A form of resistance would mean growing awareness of the impasse that comes with an oblique line connecting one subject's 'victim' position with another subject's 'aggressor' position. Another way to conceive of resistance is by imagining a horizontal line, which re-inscribes effects of recognition, in the place where the 'other of denial' (O(d)) was in the case of both subjects. Where denial was, recognition shall be. To achieve this particular horizontal line, each of the subjects would need to be capable of being in the state that I described above as oblique stillness.

A form of impasse can be driven by the analyst's guilt for not being able to help the patient sufficiently with their suffering or to 'repair' the violence of the scene of trauma. Ferenczi refers to this situation as 'superkindness' (1932a, p. 86). This is an analytic 'superperformace' which can only lead to further impasses in the transference and to blockages in the analytic process. If we keep to the scheme representing the 'dialogue of unconsciouses', in this case the dialogue is fraught because the analyst ignores or 'brackets' the plurality of the patient's psychic positions and gets stuck in regarding them as a 'victim', relating solely to the categories of denial/recognition while ignoring the all-relevant category of aggression (perhaps both in the patient and in themselves). Ultimately, this guilt-bound position of the analyst is unsustainable.

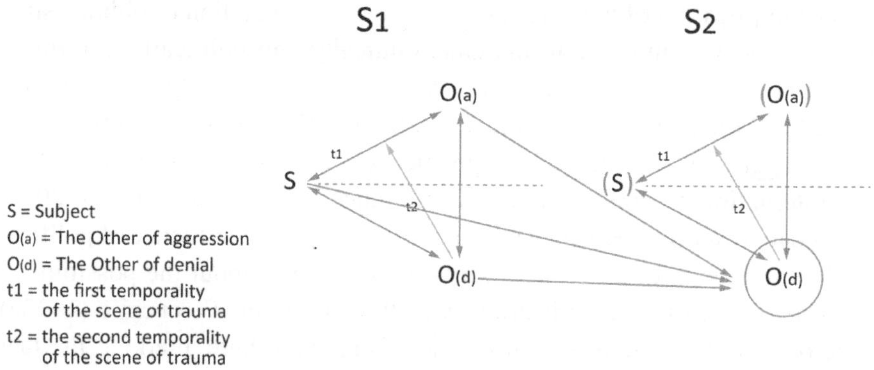

Figure 1.7 An Interpretation of the 'Superkindness' as Discussed by Sándor Ferenczi.

The state of resistance to the identification with the aggressor brings a novel psychic temporality, which I call *conditional future perfect*. This time of the verb does not exist as such: it is a necessary invention. It describes psychic actions undertaken *in the name of a time where the Other would have done less harm*. Conditional future perfect is a time of no illusions of full 'reparation' or the restoration of some state of 'integration' or 'oneness' that would have pre-existed the scene of trauma. It is a time of limited reconstruction, working with whatever exists 'on the table' of the analysis. To inhabit the world in the conditional future perfect is to ask: what if there is a way to do less harm? What would less harm have looked like then? And what might it look like now? Is there a way in which these two particular subjects can be in an entanglement where they minimise the harm they do to one another, while also engaging the grammar by which harm was done in the past?

Vignette: Charcoal on White Cotton

Liv, 50 years of age, of Afro-Brazilian descent, has recovered a long-buried memory: as a young child she was silently watching her Black grandmother, bent over the ironing board, ironing white cotton clothes with a charcoal iron. Liv then gets in touch with her child inner voice who would have observed: 'Charcoal can stain'. And also, 'This cotton cannot bear the mark of a Black woman'. We have here a figuration of the violence of the racist matrix: racialised bodies should not leave their mark nor make their inscription. Charcoal is dangerous to white cotton.

This is a completely quiet scene. No word is uttered by child-Liv – or so adult-Liv remembers the scene. The grandmother continues to iron; the granddaughter continues to watch and fear the making of a stain. Once an adult, Liv tells her White analyst about this enigmatic scene.

But let us pause for a moment on the psychoanalytic idea of a scene. Psychoanalysis is populated by many scenes: the primal scene, the scene of seduction, the scene of trauma. The scene is a fundamental unit for the organisation of psychic matter. Scenes also do not operate autonomously. We usually have a system of 'scenes', a kind of psychic scenography emerging through the *interaction* effects between different moments in time. With Freud, we saw that the traumatic consequences of the first scene are only released in the form of a symptom as a result of the retrospective action of the second scene, which has the power to reactivate or revitalise the memory traces of the first scene. The memory of the first scene lingers on in a kind of limbo or 'in storage'. It is like a foreign body. It is activated through a thread of connections and homologies.

The adult memory of the child's thought that 'This cotton cannot bear the mark of a black woman' is a complicated intersection of temporalities, referencing, I believe, many episodes of day-to-day racism, of Liv's being made to feel wrongly placed in her own skin. Retrospectively, Liv seems to have always known about the dangerous proximity of charcoal and white cotton. But this knowledge was painfully acquired through many lived episodes of racial suffering.

Here I turn to Ferenczi again, who sharpens and widens our understanding of the scene of trauma. In short, in the moment of trauma, the psyche is capable of radical forms of splitting. The psychic fragments resulting from this radical splitting acquire 'lives' of their own – they are enduring psychic formations. They have their own voices, their own associated defence mechanisms. They are enduring structures. Given the enormity of suffering experienced during the traumatic attack, psychic survival would have been impossible without the radical splitting into fragments.

So what does this mean, if we return to racist fantasies and the racist matrix? What does the possibility of radical fragmentation bring? Splitting into pieces means, as Ferenczi writes, that the 'single fragments suffer for themselves; the unbearable unification of all pain qualities and quantities does not take place'. In the racist matrix, the integration of all pain would be the equivalent of psychic death. Here, dissolving the sense of a unified perception is equated with a possibility of survival. The function of fragmentation is also that of not being there as a unified screen to be projected on, entirely available for racialised projections.

Can we imagine the ex-corporation of a scene (the reversal of its traumatic incorporation)? I believe ex-corporations are part of the radical plasticity of the psyche, acquired at the time of the trauma. The 'lives' of some of the psychic fragments include the possibility of long-distance travel ['a part of me is here and a part of me is far away'], seeing from afar ['a part of me is watching another part of me from above'], projections of a part of the ego to a far-away place ['I am both here and there'] – ultimately, many kinds of partial ex-corporations of the ego. In other words, the psyche maintains the capacity to imagine itself *away* from the racist scene.

There are important resonances here with Homi Bhabha (1984), who talks about a post-colonial subjectivity that is not constructed upon coherence and integration but upon ambivalence, alienation, and mimicry. There are also resonances with Frantz Fanon: for him, the lived experience of blackness is punctured by forms of psychical and physical pain. Images of fragmented, segmented, dismembered, shattered bodies are at the centre of the experience of having a Black body, on being in a Black skin, of inhabiting the racist matrix. As he writes, 'What else could it be for me but an amputation, an excision, a haemorrhage that spattered my whole body with black blood' (Fanon, 1986, p. 113).

*

This scene struck me, but its obliqueness invites me to take an oblique position myself in relation to what was being said. Child-Liv is watching from below. She is watching her grandmother bent over the ironing board. Exploring the fantasy further, I found out that Liv is not sure if the grandmother was being paid for her work. She was probably ironing White people's clothes for just a few pennies. The extractive line is there: racist and heteropatriarchal capitalism lives literally on the backs of its oppressed bodies. To listen to this account, one needs to lean in. To listen to this account, one needs to hear it myriads of times, as many times as the iron crossed the cotton. Charcoal on white cotton. If anything, the analysis is a process for the repeated ex-corporation of this scene, the scene of a Black woman ironing white cotton with a charcoal iron, terrified not to stain it, while her granddaughter vibrates unconsciously with the same fear. This fear binds generations into the impossibility of making a mark. So analysis aims to do the un-binding. Analysis happens in the temporality of the *conditional future perfect.* In a temporality where the Other would have done less violence.

Analysis is also a machine for sustaining and enhancing the fantasies of regurgitating, of the psychic reversal of a violent introjection. We can ask: what does regurgitating do to the racist matrix, and what does the ex-corporation of a racist scene do to the subject's state of suffering and fragmentation?

Autotomy: The Fragment Left Behind

One of the most tragic forms of autoplastic adaptation is autotomia, where the ego cuts off, disattaches and leaves behind a part of itself. It is here that Ferenczi relies on the image of the animal shedding a body part that has been wounded. Let us think of lizards cutting off their tail. In 'Psychoanalytical Observations on Tic', he writes:

> Here I will touch on the analogy of the third kind of tic, i.e. the motor discharge ('turning against one's own person', Freud), with a method of reaction that occurs in certain lower animals, which possess the capacity for 'Autotomia'. If a part of their body is painfully stimulated they let the part concerned 'fall' in the true sense of the word by severing it from the rest of their body by the help of certain specialized muscular

> actions; others (like certain worms) even fall into several small pieces (they 'burst asunder', as it were, from fury). Even the biting off of a painful limb is said to occur.
>
> (Ferenczi, 1921, p. 160)

In one of the entries in the *Clinical Diary*, Ferenczi brings another vignette on animal behaviour, where the adaptation to the anticipation of unbearable pain and complete submission is suicide:

> As an analogy I refer to a reliable account of an Indian friend, a hunter. He saw how a falcon attacked a little bird; as it approached, the little bird started to tremble and, after a few seconds of trembling, flew straight into the falcon's open beak and was swallowed up. The anticipation of certain death appears to be such torment that by comparison actual death is a relief.
>
> (Ferenczi, 1932a, p. 179)

Ferenczi derives crucial metapsychological reflections from these images. In the first example, on autotomia, we see 'an archaic prototype of the components of the masochistic instinct' (Ferenczi, 1921, p. 161). In the second, we see the limits of passivity and a certain primacy given to activity, in that an active death is preferred to the anticipation of complete surrender to the aggressor. In a fragment on 'Trauma and Anxiety', Ferenczi strengthens the same idea: 'Self-destruction as releasing some anxiety is preferred to silent toleration' (Ferenczi, 1931a, p. 249). It appears that the easiest to break apart is the conscious system, responsible for the integration of mental images into a unit. Ultimately, splitting is an act that is more readily available to the psyche than we are used to considering. Structurally, it seems that the fragment that is severed in the process of autotomy is not preserved in a modified form in the superego but is irretrievably lost. In terms of psychic temporality, to be irretrievably lost means to exist in a kind of *non-time*, or outside of a sequence, or of a scene structured by different times, or of a significant and structuring clash of times, as is the case in the Freudian *Nachträglichkeit.*

Teratoma: The Buried Fragment

The catastrophe, as we saw above, is *both destructive and creative.* How can we further make sense of this tension between radical destruction and radical creativity? A curious formation appears in Ferenczi's work precisely at this difficult crossing: it is the *teratoma* – the fruit of one of his medical analogies, where he compares the growth of a complicated (cancerous) tumour with a psychic phenomenon. In his 1929 paper 'The Principle of Relaxation and Neocatharsis', Ferenczi notes:

> For it is no mere poetic licence to compare the mind of the neurotic to a double malformation, something like the so-called teratoma which harbours in a hidden part of its body fragments of a twin-being which has never developed. No reasonable person would refuse to surrender such a teratoma to the surgeon's knife, if the existence of the whole individual were threatened.
>
> (Ferenczi, 1929, p. 123)

Georg Groddeck (1923) used a similar term in a literary context when he spoke of 'horror stories': teratomae were a particular type of monster, either constructed from parts of different bodies, like Frankenstein, or the result of fantasy and the transformations of the body that fantasy brings (Stanton, 1991, p. 174). Medically, the teratoma is a tumour, made up of various types of tissue that may or may not be cancerous. The implications of Ferenczian teratomae are, however, much deeper. Ferenczi argues that in some cases of neurosis the greater part of the personality becomes a teratoma, while the task of adaptation to reality falls upon the (smaller) fragment of the personality that was spared. I believe the work of the psychoanalytic process is to deal with this very disproportion, where the deadened 'twin-being' occupies most of the psychic space. This is perhaps the Ferenczian uncanny: a meeting with the twin-inside. The act of the (Ferenczian) narcissist is that of denying the very existence of the teratoma.

As early as 1908, in a text on 'Psycho-Analysis and Education', Ferenczi was already noting the existence in the unconscious of a parasitic double of the conscious self 'whose natural egotism and tendency for unscrupulous wish-fulfilment represents the dark phantom, the negative of all the good and beautiful on which the higher consciousness prides itself' (Ferenczi, 1908a, p. 287). This type of split psychic functioning creates 'introspective blindness' which is preserved through moralising education. Through the 'prohibiting and deterring commands of moralising education' (Ferenczi, 1908a), the person settles into a state akin to that of hypnosis, with diminished mental energies flowing in the conscious part of the ego and with considerably impaired capacity for action. What is remarkable here is that, in contrast with the writings of Melanie Klein, projection is much less readily available to the psyche. It is often the case that internal 'badness' (especially that resulting from various facets of the identification with the aggressor) is retained in the psyche, and while it is retained it also generates structural modifications of the psyche which require important metapsychological revisions. This is why Ferenczi feels the need to name this psychic place, which he refers to as an internal 'parasite' at an earlier point in his works. Two decades later, this parasitic psychic place will become the 'teratoma'.

I believe that the 'teratoma' is involved in the development of a particular aspect of the superego. In 'Fantasies on a Biological Model of Super-Ego Formation', Ferenczi returns to a scene of devouring and swallowing whole that he attributes to the identification with the aggressor (Ferenczi, 1930c, p. 228). We discussed above this sort of incorporation of an unmetabolised whole. It is important to stress that the 'scene of devouring' is quite fluid and circulates freely in the psyche: from the act of having swallowed the aggressor whole, the psyche easily produces fantasies of having swallowed somebody else and of having swallowed itself. The twin-being of the teratoma is also created through a fantasy of having swallowed oneself. What develops from here is a kind of 'mad superego' that is not an introjection of a person or of an aspect of a person, but of a *scene*. What is incessantly replayed in this scene is the encounter between an 'over-great (fat) aggressor' and 'a much smaller, weaker person, oppressed and dominated by the aggressor' (Ferenczi, 1930c). This is the fundamental asymmetry that we marked above in the discussion of the identification with the aggressor.

After taking this journey with the teratoma, I return to tentacular knowledge. This 'dark' creation, this monstrous agglomeration of psychic fragments of different sorts can only be apprehended by a tactile eye. To put it in Goodfield's terms, 'if you really want to understand about a tumor, you've got to be a tumor' (1981, p. 213).

The teratoma is an instance of radical psychic plasticity. This means that sometimes parts of the organism can appear dead, but they retain the capacity to build a new psychic formation or fragment out of their own detritus. This is an important implicit conversation that Ferenczi has with Freud on the place of the death drive, marking that 'organisms are not so eager to die' (1924, p. 90). Indeed, this is not, in my reading, an abandonment of the death drive as a clinical-theoretical construct. It is instead a curiosity about the many forms that the life drive can and does take. In *Thalassa*, an image that Ferenczi ponders over is that of a 'protective' bladder, membrane, vesicle, pustule or 'place of abode' filled with fluid (1924, p. 64). Such protective creations are directly implicated in psychic survival at the time of catastrophe, and they count as a manifestation of the life drive.

*

In this first part of the book, I wished to create a montage that takes the reader into the atmosphere of living among fragments, scraps, detritus but also new growths, protective membranes and contagions. While wondering about the psychic life of fragments, psychoanalysis itself is transformed. I understand this transformation as a constellation of three different modalities of psychoanalytic attention. Firstly, it is a psychoanalysis of scars, held together by a vocabulary of wounds and scar-tissues and which has a 'traumatophilic' inclination. Here, the attention goes to a scar-tissue resulting from the encounter with the Other, out of which both memory and the ego are made. Secondly, it is a psychoanalysis of organs, animated by an interest in radical plasticity, an attention to the surprising modes of psychic splitting that result from the scene of trauma, and to the 'semifluid' bodies and organs that reshape, retract, and grow new parts. Here, the guiding question is 'what can an organ *do*?' or 'what can a fragment *do*?'. Thirdly, it is an eventful psychoanalysis, holding on to an interest in catastrophe and trauma. Here, the images that predominate are those of fractures, splits, atomisations, pulverisations, but also new organs and expansions. As I have shown, catastrophe is not a single, unitary event but a *scene* where several elements hold together in relation and interact, often in a violent manner. As a result, new structures and psychic positions are formed, while some old ones are destroyed. To approach the scene of trauma, I paid attention to oblique lines, un-common transversal trajectories, orientations that are from below or from above, which happen in an asymmetric encounter between small and large, between powerless and overpowering, between fixed and movable.

Notes

1 I thank Matt ffytche for formulating this question in a commentary to the book I co-authored with Jenny Willner and Jakob Staberg (Soreanu et al., 2023).

2 For Klein's (1946) description of splitting processes, her 'Notes on Some Schizoid Mechanisms' paper is of particular importance. As she writes, 'From the beginning the destructive impulse is turned against the object and is first expressed in phantasied oral-sadistic attacks on the mother's breast, which soon develop into onslaughts on her body by all sadistic means. The persecutory fears arising from the infant's oral-sadistic

impulses to rob the mother's body of its good contents, and from the anal-sadistic impulses to put his excrements into her (including the desire to enter her body in order to control her from within) are of great importance for the development of paranoia and schizophrenia' (Klein, 1946, p. 2).

3 As Klein states: 'In my view, the splitting of the ego, by which the superego is formed, comes about as a consequence of conflict in the ego, engendered by the polarity of the two instincts. This conflict is increased by their projection as well as by the resulting introjection of good and bad objects. The ego, supported by the internalized good object and strengthened by the identification with it, projects a portion of the death instinct into that part of itself which it has split off—a part which thus comes to be in opposition to the rest of the ego and forms the basis of the super-ego. Accompanying this deflection of a portion of the death instinct is a deflection of that portion of the life instinct which is fused with it. Along with these deflections, parts of the good and bad objects are split off from the ego into the super-ego. The super-ego thus acquires both protective and threatening qualities. As the process of integration—present from the beginning in both the ego and the super-ego—goes on, the death instinct is bound, up to a point, by the super-ego. In the process of binding, the death instinct influences the aspects of the good objects contained in the super-ego, with the result that the action of the super-ego ranges from restraint of hate and destructive impulses, protection of the good object and self-criticism, to threats, inhibitory complaints and persecution. The super-ego—being bound up with the good object and even striving for its preservation—comes close to the actual good mother who feeds the child and takes care of it, but since the super-ego is also under the influence of the death instinct, it partly becomes the representative of the mother who frustrates the child, and its prohibitions and accusations arouse anxiety' (Klein, 1958, p. 240).

4 For other voices in the phenomenology of race, see Gordon (1995); Macey (1999); Alcoff (1999).

5 In the original, in Portuguese: 'A possibilidade de percepções de transmissões mudas são, a meu ver, limitadas pela posição clássica, do analista. A 'posição diagonal' do analista, quer dizer, o fato de estar ele sentado atrás e ao lado do paciente, permite melhor do que a posição clássica, à observações de comunicações mudas expressas pela mímica, pelos gestos e tudo o que se exprime de maneira óbvia pelo motor. Acho que a 'posição diagonal', permite ao paciente tanto quanto ele necessita, perceber e olhar o analista; como possibilita ao analista a melhor percepção de transmissões mudas. Veja a concepção de Th. Benedek (sentar-se atrás do paciente pode corresponder a uma fuga do analista)' (Kemper, 1962).

References

Ahmed, S. (2006). *Queer Phenomenology: Orientations, Objects, Others*. Durham, NC: Duke University Press.

Alcoff, L. M. (1999). Towards a phenomenology of racial embodiment. *Radical Philosophy*, 95: 15–26.

Bálint, A. (1943). Identification. *International Journal of Psychoanalysis,* 24: 97–107.

Baraitser, L. (2017). *Enduring Time*. London: Bloomsbury.

Baraitser, L. (2023). Passivity and gender: Psychical inertia and maternal stillness. *International Journal of Psychoanalysis*, 104(5): 912–926.

Benjamin, J. (2018). *Beyond Doer and Done to: Recognition Theory, Intersubjectivity and the Third.* London & New York, NY: Routledge.

Berlant, L., & Warner, M. (2005). Sex in public. In: M. Warner (ed.), *Public and Counterpublics* (pp. 187–208). New York, NY: Zone Books.

Bhabha, H. K. (1984). Of mimicry and man the ambivalence of colonial discourse. 28: 125–133.
Birksted-Breen, D. (2003). Time and the après-coup. *International Journal of Psychoanalysis*, 84: 1501–1515.
Bragin, M. (2007). Knowing terrible things: Engaging survivors of extreme violence in treatment. *Clinical Social Work Journal*, 35(4): 229–236.
Castoriadis, C. (1987). *The Imaginary Institution of Society*. Cambridge: Polity Press.
Castoriadis, C. (1989a). Done and to be done. In: D. A. Curtis (ed.), *The Castoriadis Reader* (pp. 361–417). Oxford: Blackwell.
Castoriadis, C. (1989b). The state of the subject today. *Thesis Eleven*, 24: 5–43.
Cavarero, A. (2016). *Inclinations: A Critique of Rectitude* (transl. A. Minervini & A. Sitze). Stanford, CA: Stanford University Press.
Dahl, G. (2010). The two time vectors of *Nachträglichkeit* in the development of Ego organization: Significance of the concept for the symbolization of nameless traumas and anxieties. *International Journal of Psychoanalysis*, 91: 727–744.
Dahms, I. (2023). Maternal inclinations, queer orientations, common occupation. *Critical Horizons*, 24(2): 147–163.
Faimberg, H. (2007). A plea for a broader concept of *Nachträglichkeit*. *Psychoanalytic Quarterly*, 76: 1221–1240.
Fanon, F. (1986). *Black Skin, White Masks* (transl. by C. L. Markmann). London: Pluto Press.
Ferenczi, S. (1908a). Psycho-analysis and education. In: *Final Contributions to the Problems and Methods of Psycho-analysis* (transl. by E. Mosbacher, pp. 280–290). London: Karnac, 1994.
Ferenczi, S. (1908b). The analytic conception of the psycho-neuroses. In: *Further Contributions to the Theory and Technique of Psycho-analysis* (transl. by J. I. Suttie, pp. 15–30). London: Karnac, 1994.
Ferenczi, S. (1909). Introjection and transference. In: *First Contributions to Psycho-analysis* (transl. by E. Jones, pp 35–93). London: Karnac, 1994.
Ferenczi, S. (1912). On epileptic fits. *Final Contributions to the Problems and Methods of Psycho-analysis* (transl. by E. Mosbacher, pp. 197–204). London: Karnac, 1994.
Ferenczi, S. (1913). Stages in the development of the sense of reality. In: *First Contributions to Psycho-analysis* (transl. by E. Jones, pp. 213–239). London: Karnac, 1994.
Ferenczi, S. (1915). The analysis of comparisons. In: *Further Contributions to the Theory and Technique of Psycho-analysis* (transl. by J. I. Suttie, pp. 397–407). London: Karnac, 1994.
Ferenczi, S. (1919). The phenomena of hysterical materialization. In: *Further Contributions to the Theory and Technique of Psycho-analysis* (transl. by J. I. Suttie, pp. 89–104). London: Karnac, 1994.
Ferenczi, S. (1921). The symbolism of the bridge. In: *Further Contributions to the Theory and Technique of Psycho-analysis* (transl. by J. I. Suttie, pp. 352–356). London: Karnac, 1994.
Ferenczi, S. (1922a). Psycho-analysis and the mental disorders of general paralysis of the insane. In: *Final Contributions to the Problems and Methods of Psycho-analysis* (transl. by E. Mosbacher, pp. 351–370). London: Karnac, 1994.
Ferenczi, S. (1922b). Freud's 'group psychology and the analysis of the ego'. In: *Final Contributions to the Problems and Methods of Psycho-analysis* (transl. by E. Mosbacher, pp. 371–376). London: Karnac.

Ferenczi, S. (1926). The problem of acceptance of unpleasant ideas–advances in knowledge of the sense of reality. In: *Further Contributions to the Theory and Technique of Psychoanalysis* (transl. by J. I. Suttie, pp. 366–379). London: Karnac, 1994.

Ferenczi, S. (1929). The principle of relaxation and neocatharsis. In: *Final Contributions to the Problems and Methods of Psycho-analysis* (transl. by E. Mosbacher, pp. 108–125). London: Karnac, 1994.

Ferenczi, S. (1930a). Autoplastic and alloplastic adaptation. In: *Final Contributions to the Problems and Methods of Psycho-analysis* (transl. by E. Mosbacher, p. 221). London: Karnac, 1994.

Ferenczi, S. (1930b). Each adaptation is preceded by an inhibited attempt at splitting. In: *Final Contributions to the Problems and Methods of Psycho-analysis* (transl. by E. Mosbacher, p. 220). London: Karnac, 1994.

Ferenczi, S. (1930c). Fantasies on a biological model of super-ego formation. In: *Final Contributions to the Problems and Methods of Psycho-analysis* (transl. by E. Mosbacher, pp. 227–230). London: Karnac, 1994.

Ferenczi, S. (1930d). Trauma and striving for health. In: *Final Contributions to the Problems and Methods of Psycho-analysis* (transl. by E. Mosbacher, pp. 230–231). London: Karnac, 1994.

Ferenczi, S. (1931a). Child-analysis in the analysis of adults. In: *Final Contributions to the Problems and Methods of Psycho-analysis* (transl. by E. Mosbacher, pp. 126–142). London: Karnac, 1994.

Ferenczi, S. (1931b). On the revision of the interpretation of dreams. In: *Final Contributions to the Problems and Methods of Psycho-analysis* (transl. by E. Mosbacher, pp. 238–243). London: Karnac, 1994.

Ferenczi, S. (1931c). The birth of intellect. In: *Final Contributions to the Problems and Methods of Psycho-analysis* (transl. by E. Mosbacher, pp. 244–246). London: Karnac, 1994.

Ferenczi, S. (1932a). *The Clinical Diary of Sándor Ferenczi*, ed. by J. Dupont (transl. by M. Bálint & N. Z. Jackson). Cambridge, MA: Harvard University Press, 1995.

Ferenczi, S. (1932b). On shock. In: *Final Contributions to the Problems and Methods of Psycho-analysis* (transl. by E. Mosbacher, E., pp. 253–254). London: Karnac, 1994.

Ferenczi, S. (1933). The confusion of tongues between adults and the child. In: *Final Contributions to the Problems and Methods of Psycho-analysis* (transl. by E. Mosbacher, pp. 156–167). London: Karnac, 1994.

Ferenczi, S. (1924). *Thalassa. A Theory of Genitality* (transl. by H. A. Bunker). London & New York, NY: Karnac, 1989.

Fletcher, J. (2013). *Freud and the Scene of Trauma*. New York, NY: Fordham University Press.

Frankel, J. (1998). Ferenczi's trauma theory. *American Journal of Psychoanalysis*, 58(1): 41–61.

Frankel, J. (2015) The persistent sense of being bad: The moral dimension of the identification with the aggressor. In: A. Harris & S. Kuchuck (eds), *The Legacy of Sándor Ferenczi: From Ghost to Ancestor* (pp. 204–222). London & New York, NY: Routledge.

Freud, A. (1936). *The Ego and the Mechanisms of Defence*. London: Hogarth Press.

Freud, S. (1909). Notes upon a case of obsessional neurosis (Rat Man). In: *Standard Edition* (Vol. 10, pp. 151–318). London: Hogarth Press.

Freud, S. (1913). Totem and tabu. In: *Standard Edition* (Vol. 13, pp. vii–162). London: Hogarth Press.

Freud, S. (1915). Instincts and their vicissitudes. In: *Standard Edition* (Vol. 14, pp. 109–140). London: Hogarth Press.
Freud, S. (1921). Group psychology and the analysis of the ego. In: *Standard Edition* (Vol. 18, pp. 67–143). London: Hogarth Press.
Freud, S. (1938). Splitting of the Ego in the process of defence. In: *Standard Edition* (Vol. 23, pp. 271–278). London: Hogarth Press.
Gil, J. (1997). *Metamorfoses do corpo*. Lisboa: Relógio D'Água.
Goodfield, J. (1981). *An Imagined World*. New York, NY: Harper and Rowe.
Gordon, L. R. (1995). *Fanon and the Crisis of European Man: An Essay on Philosophy and the Human Sciences*. London: Routledge.
Groddeck, G. (1923). *The Book of the It* (transl. by V. M. E.Collins). New York, NY: Funk & Wagnalls Company.
Guattari, F. (2011). *The Machinic Unconscious: Essays in Schizoanalysis* (transl. by T. Adkins). Los Angeles, CA: Semiotext(e).
Gumbs, A. P. (2020a). *Undrowned: Black Feminist Lessons from Marine Mammals*. Chico, CA: AK Press.
Gumbs, A. P. (2020b). *Dub: Finding Ceremony*. Durham, NC: Duke University Press.
Haraway, D. J. (2016). *Staying with the Trouble: Making Kin in the Chthulucene*. Durham, NC: Duke University Press.
Hristeva, G. (2013). 'Uterus loquitur': Trauma and the human organism in Ferenczi's 'physiology of pleasure'. *American Journal of Psychoanalysis*, 73(4): 339–352.
Huidobro, V. (2003). *Altazor* (transl. by E. Weinberger). Middletown, CT: Wesleyan University Press.
Kemper, K. (1962). *A interpretação aludida: Sua relação com as vivências e comunicações pré-verbais*. Unpublished manuscript.
Klein, M. (1933). The early development of conscience in the child. In: *The Writings of Melanie Klein* (Vol. 1, pp. 248–257). London: Hogarth Press.
Klein, M. (1946). Notes on some schizoid mechanisms. In: *The Writings of Melanie Klein* (Vol. 3, pp. 1–24). London: Hogarth Press.
Klein, M. (1955). On identification. In: *The Writings of Melanie Klein* (Vol. 3, pp. 141–175). London: Hogarth Press.
Klein, M. (1958). On the development of mental functioning. In: *The Writings of Melanie Klein* (Vol. 3, pp. 236–246). London: Hogarth Press.
Kristeva, J. (1984). *Revolution in Poetic Language*. New York, NY: Columbia University Press.
Kristeva, J. (2000). *The Sense and non-sense of Revolt: The Powers and Limits of Psychoanalysis*. New York, NY: Columbia University Press.
Laplanche, J. (1997). The theory of seduction and the problem of the other. *The International Journal of Psychoanalysis*, 78: 653–666.
Laplanche, J. (1998). *Notes sur l'après-coup* [Paper presented at the Conference on psychoanalytical intracultural and intercultural dialogue. International Psychoanalytical Association, Paris, 27–29 July].
Laplanche, J. (1999a). *Entre Seduction et Inspiration: L'homme*. Paris: Presses Universitaires de France.
Laplanche, J. (1999b). Sublimation and/or Inspiration. *New Formations*, 48: 2002–2003.
Laplanche, J. (1999c). *Essays on Otherness*. London & New York, NY: Routledge.
Lénárd, K., & Tényi, T. (2003). Ferenczi's concept on trauma, connected with the Katonadolog – 'Soldiers can take it' concept. *International Forum of Psycho-Analysis*, 12(1): 22–29.

Lévi-Strauss, C. (1961). *Tristes Tropiques* (transl. by J. Russell). New York, NY: Criterion Books.

Macey, D. (1999). Fanon, phenomenology, race. *Radical Philosophy*, 95: 8–14.

Mentz, S. (2015). *Shipwreck Modernity: Ecologies of Globalization, 1550–1719.* Minneapolis, MN: University of Minnesota Press.

Oliner, M. (2013). 'Non-represented' mental states. In: H. B. Levine, G. S. Reed, & D. Scarfone (eds), *Unrepresented States and the Construction of Meaning: Clinical and Theoretical Contributions* (pp. 152–171). London: Karnac.

Picasso, P. (1945). Found objects. In: H. B. Chipp (ed.), *Theories of Modern Art.* Berkeley & Los Angeles, CA: University of California Press, 1968.

Saketopoulou, A. (2023). *Sexuality Beyond Consent: Risk, Race, Traumatophilia.* New York, NY: New York University Press.

Scarfone, D. (2019). The feminine, the analyst and the child theorist. *International Journal of Psychoanalysis,* 100(3): 567–575.

Sharpe, C. (2016). *In the Wake: On Blackness and Being.* Durham, NC: Duke University Press.

Soreanu, R. (2018a). The psychic life of fragments: Splitting from Ferenczi to Klein. *American Journal of Psychoanalysis*, 78(4): 421–444.

Soreanu, R. (2018b). *Working-Through Collective Wounds: Trauma, Denial, Recognition in the Brazilian Uprising.* London: Palgrave Macmillan.

Soreanu, R., Staberg, J., & Willner, J. (2023). *Ferenczi Dialogues: On Trauma and Catastrophe*. Leuven: Leuven University Press.

Staberg, J. (2023). Instead of language: Confusion. Sigmund Freud/Sándor Ferenczi. In: R. Soreanu, J. Staberg, & J. Willner (eds), *Ferenczi Dialogues: On Trauma and Catastrophe* (pp. 23–71). Leuven: Leuven University Press.

Stanton, M. (1991). *Sándor Ferenczi: Reconsidering Active Intervention.* London: Free Association Books.

Vyrgioti, M. (2021). Freud and the cannibal: Vignettes from psychoanalysis' colonial history. In: S. Bar-Haim, E. S. Coles, & H. Tyson (eds), *Wild Analysis: From the Couch to Cultural and Political Life* (pp. 67–81). London: Routledge.

Willner, J. (2023). Catastrophes and genitality: Ferenczi's *Thalassa* and the politics of bioanalysis. In: R. Soreanu, J. Staberg, & J. Willner (eds), *Ferenczi Dialogues: On Trauma and Catastrophe* (pp. 91–130). Leuven: Leuven University Press.

Wilson, E. (2015). *Gut Feminism.* Durham & London: Duke University Press.

Zygouris, R. (1999). *Pulsões de vida* (transl. by C. Koltai & C. L. Valladares). São Paulo: Escuta.

Chapter 2

Repetition, Reliving and the Drives

What Was Lost in 'Beyond the Pleasure Principle'?

Freud's 1920 text 'Beyond the Pleasure Principle' marks one of the most significant breaks in his thought. It is in this text that Freud inaugurates the idea of the death drive. In what follows, I ponder some of the unspoken losses that psychoanalytic theory has suffered with this ground-breaking text. This is not to say, however, that the theoretical ramifications of introducing the death drive/life drive pairing are few. The clinical implications of being able to speak in terms of the death drive are outstanding. Here, I diverge from voices arguing that we can do without the idea of the death drive in clinical work (De Masi, 2015), or that the death drive can be treated as an unaccomplished and ambiguous metaphor for human aggressiveness (Frank, 2015).

After Alfred Adler and Carl Jung had left the theoretical domain constituted around the libido theory, Freud had very high stakes in affirming and preserving it. But, curiously enough, in 'Beyond the Pleasure Principle' he questions the libido theory as he had proposed it so far. This break was hard to handle even in Freud's circle of the time. Freud's followers (Karl Abraham and Max Eitingon, for instance) remained somewhat puzzled when confronted with Freud's radical revision and with the discovery of the death drive. Some of them attributed it to a philosophical disposition in Freud or to a kind of cultural pessimism of the time which had little to do to metapsychology (Young-Bruehl, 2011; Frank, 2015). But the death drive proved to be more than a temporary philosophical leaning in dark times. It became the core of a revised metapsychology.

Freud starts from a newly observed kind of repetition – or a repetition he is now able to look at from a new perspective – which brings him to the hypothesis that there is something akin to a death drive operating in the

DOI: 10.4324/9781032715926-3

psyche. The repetition he speaks of is not directly in service to the pleasure principle. He discusses repetition in traumatic dreams and in children's games (the famous 'Fort/Da' game). In both of these examples, the dreamer or the child playing cannot derive pleasure from their repeated act. This means that there is another force organising these acts (or compulsions to repeat): Freud will give this force the name of 'death drive'.

Despite the novel proposition of the death drive, 'Beyond the Pleasure Principle' is a text traversed by contradictions, tensions, shifts and ambivalences. The death drive is defined throughout the text in different keys: as auto-aggression; then as organic elasticity; as inertia; and as the compulsion to repeat. As Philippe Van Haute and Herman Westerink (2022, 2024) have shown, Freud oscillates between monism and dualism. They understand this text as traversed by disparate approaches and as consisting of separate emerging parts. Yet there seems to be no 'beyond' the pleasure principle, as all drives seek the reduction of tension and are thus conservative.

Freud's 'Beyond the Pleasure Principle' has enduring effects on contemporary clinical imaginaries, which are still dominated by the forms of the death drive. I read this as a bias towards the death drive, its repetitions, compulsions and forms of unlinking. Jakob Staberg (2023, 2024) offers a reading of 'Beyond the Pleasure Principle' and its life drive/death drive construction as part of a discourse intrinsic to modernity, 'hovering on the verge of catastrophe in which nature and death are given new meaning within the field of culture' (Staberg, 2023, p. 30). 'Beyond the Pleasure Principle' is thus a text-event, not only because it introduces a radical rupture in the domain of metapsychology, but also because it articulates a kind of call to the field, summoning us to take a position (Grubrich-Simitis, 1993; May, 2015; Staberg, 2023, 2024). Staberg (2023, p. 30) sees this Freudian writing as 'an alien body in metapsychology that subsequent psychoanalytic theory has sought either to incorporate or displace'. Within this field of insistence and return to the 'foreign object' of the death drive, our task in this chapter is to follow Ferenczi's orientations (and disorientations) in relation to the death drive, and the ramifications these orientations have for psychoanalytic theory and practice today.

In what follows, I ask: what do we lose in the radical revision in 'Beyond the Pleasure Principle', and what can still be imagined in the horizon of the drives? I argue that there are two things lost in 'Beyond the Pleasure Principle', and I believe they are subtly interrelated. Firstly, Freud does not construct theoretical 'inheritors' for what, until 1920, he referred to as 'the ego instincts'. There is something akin to a suspension. The death drive fully dominates the scene and we never come to see an articulation of ego-preservative instincts.

Secondly, there is a strong link in Freudian thinking between the compulsion to repeat and the death drive. By focusing on the metapsychological propositions of Sándor Ferenczi, I aim to pluralise our thinking on repetition. This extends to a rereading of the Freudian version of deferred action or afterwardsness [*Nachträglichkeit*] and of the temporalities of the psyche. I discuss a new psychic time, the time of reliving. Through this idea, Ferenczi gave a whole different meaning than Freud did to the series repetition/remembering/reliving. I trace its genealogy in the scene of trauma and I connect it to the event of survival. I then trace the way the time of reliving operates in the consulting room, through moments that Ferenczi calls 'neo-catharsis'. I construct a clinical vignette to further imagine the time of reliving.

Finally, I explore Ferenczi's ideas on 'the feminine principle', showing how it constitutes an important intervention in the sphere of the drives, which has clinical relevance in the contemporary clinic. Ferenczi articulates a vocabulary in which terms such as conciliation, endurance of suffering, selflessness, appeasement, adaptation, renunciation, self-denial and compromise, percolate and are arranged in a surprising way, with a direct relation to Ferenczi's trauma theory. The feminine principle brings a rethinking of the reality principle, a re-evaluation of the duality of the drives and of the unexplored forms of the life drive. The value of this 'life drive imaginary' emerges, however, as something other than a naïve vitalism or a generic, optimistic image of the prevalence of life over death. In *The Clinical Diary,* Ferenczi presents us with a particular modification to the sphere of the death drive/life drive dualism: he renames them the 'drive of self-assertion' and the 'drive of conciliation'. The 'selflessness' he evokes includes the 'selflessness' of organs: it emerges in relation to the scene of trauma, and it ultimately describes a complex psychic state that considers otherness and the relationship to the environment. The 'drive for conciliation' expresses the fact that, in order to survive as any sort of individuality, one needs to practice a kind of politics of self-limitation. These ideas on 'the feminine principle' are tied in with a revision of conceptions of genitality. Ferenczi invites us to democratise forms of erotism: he has in mind a clever combination of mechanisms of pleasure, and rich mixtures and transpositions of the erotic in psychic life.

The Lost Inheritors of the Ego Instincts

What happens to the lost ego instincts in psychoanalytic theory? Elisabeth Young-Bruehl (2011) speaks in strong terms, using the formulation, 'the trauma of lost love in psychoanalysis' and accounting for the text 'Beyond the Pleasure Principle' as having a traumatic and inhibiting quality. In this text, as noted above, Freud was marking a change of theoretical route, but underneath this was an ardent wish for further development and integration of his previous formulations.

There are significant consequences of focusing on the death drive and of postulating that the pleasure principle operates in service of the death drive. As I show below, a form of love remains unaccounted for, and it is ultimately lost to psychoanalytic theory.

In his 1911 paper 'Formulations on the Two Principles of Mental Functioning', Freud (1911) articulates a conceptual pair: pleasure principle [*Lustprinzip*] and reality principle [*Realitätsprinzip*]. As long as the newborn is adequately cared for, the *Lustprinzip* operates without much constraint. It produces tensions and excitations that the newborn is able to discharge via hallucinations (attached to memories of past pleasures). The *Realitätsprinzip*, by contrast, has hunger as its prototype and, in a brief formulation, refers to tensions and excitations that need an object (distinct from mere hallucinations – for instance, real food) in order to be discharged. The 1911 theoretical 'house' is thus governed by two drives – the libidinal one and the ego-instinctual one.

Here, I draw attention to the fact that surprisingly little happened, in theoretical terms, to the ego-instinctual drive (or the self-preservative drive) in the period between 1911 and 1920. In 1920, the ego instinct was finally discarded. No inheritors were constructed for it while Freud moved to a new theoretical house. In 'Beyond the Pleasure Principle', all that Freud (1920) has to say about the ego-preservative instincts is contained in a short reference on page 10, where he mentions that the *Realitätsprinzip* is 'under the influence of the ego's instincts of self-preservation'.

It is the Budapest School that preserved and elaborated the idea of self-preservative drives or ego instincts as valuable in themselves. It is also the thinkers of the Budapest School who saw that psychoanalysis could not proceed without a philosophy of love and a moral-political theory (Young-Bruehl, 2011, p. 261). In the works of the Budapest School, we can encounter a metapsychological expression of the ancient Greek insistence on the fact that although *eros* is a contrasting force to *philia*, the two are also strongly intertwined. *Philia* refers to all bonds with living beings, without which survival and life in common are impossible to envisage. As Young-Bruehl (2011, p. 253) stresses, it refers to the affections and loves that exist between parents and children, between friends, between fellow citizens discussing the fate of the polity, between apprentices and their mentors. This return to *eros* and *philia* does not mean making this ancient Greek idea a replacement for metapsychology. It can instead be seen as a sub-stratum for metapsychological formulations.

In his *Thalassa*, Ferenczi (1924) talks about a form of self-preservative instinct that presents itself as a longing to return to the womb. Proposing an extended analogy between phylogenesis and ontogenesis, he articulates his own version of an origin myth which begins in the depth of the sea and manifests as a wish to return to that oceanic environment. While creating this origin myth, Ferenczi does not, however, lose sight of the sexual drives; and he also accepts a version of the death-instinct theory. Such an articulation stands as proof that there is no necessary exclusion between working with an idea of a self-preservative instinct and working with an idea of the death drive.

In the 1929 paper 'The Unwelcome Child and His Death Instinct', Ferenczi overtly recognises the importance of the Freudian life drive-death drive dualism:

> Since the epoch-making work of Freud on the irreducible instinctual foundations of everything organic (in 'Beyond the Pleasure Principle') we have become accustomed to look upon all the phenomena of life, including those of mental life, as in the last resort a mixture of the forms of expression of the two fundamental instincts: the life and the death instinct.
>
> (1929b, p. 102)

Still, Ferenczi (idem, p. 103) speaks of the 'genesis of unconscious self-destructive trends' (manifested in circulatory and respiratory disturbances, in asthma, emaciation without anatomical causes, or glottal spasms that lead to self-strangulation). The genesis is in the child's having been unwelcome to the family – or at first received well and later 'dropped'. The death drive is thus not seen to operate in an autonomous way, but it is mediated by suffering and trauma, especially the trauma of an early lack of affect. In my view, Ferenczi here outlines the relationship between the operation of the death drive and the strength of the ego. He states that the death drive is more forceful in the early stages of life, as 'the infant is [...] much closer to individual non-being' and '[s]lipping back into this non-being might therefore come much more easily to children' (idem, p. 105). The frail young ego is in much more danger of giving up on life and giving in to self-destructive tendencies. A strengthened adult ego is closer to the life drive.

It is important to note that in a series of notes in his *Clinical Diary* (in the entry of 13 August 1932), Ferenczi comes to doubt the plausibility of the death drive and affirms the insufficient exploration of the life drive.

> Even science is 'passionate' when it sees and recognises only selfish instincts. The natural urge to *share feelings of pleasure* following the corresponding normal satiation, and nature's principle of harmony, are not sufficiently recognized.
> The idea of the death instinct foes too far, is already tinged with sadism; drive to rest [*Ruhetrieb*] and SHARING (communication [*Mit-teilung*], *sharing*) of 'excessive' accumulations of pleasure *and* unpleasure is the reality, or it was when not artificially – traumatically – disturbed.
> BEING ALONE leads to splitting.
> The presence of someone with whom one can share and communicate joy and sorrow (love and understanding) can HEAL the trauma.
> Personality is reassembled '*healed*' (like 'glue').
>
> (Ferenczi, 1932a, pp. 200–201)

Avello (1998) interprets the connection Ferenczi makes between the idea of the death drive and sadism as a disavowal of the death drive. Indeed, if we autonomise and biologise the functioning of the death drive, there is little recognition of the traumatogenic actions performed by an aggressor. Yet I believe Ferenczi's diary entry cannot be taken as a fully fledged refutation of the death drive: instead, it is a statement on the insufficient theoretical energies that have gone into understanding the life drive and the *Philia*, explicitly marked here as sharing and communicating pleasure.

Perhaps Ferenczi's most original contribution to imagining inheritors for Freud's lost ego-preservative drives is his theorisation around 'Orpha'. I will discuss this feminine Orpheus at length in the next chapter. For now, I note that Orpha is a strange fragment of the psyche, resulting from the splitting process that happens in traumatic moments. Orpha is the form that the organising life instincts take at the time of the trauma, precisely when the enormity of suffering has brought a renunciation of any expectation of external help. As Ferenczi notes in his *Clinical Diary*: '[t]he absent external help [...] is replaced by the creation of a more ancient substitute' (1932a, p. 105). Orpha is a sort of 'guardian angel' or a healing agent. It is capable of unusual, minute calculations around what it would mean to continue living. It can ask and answer questions: how many heartbeats per second to continue living? It thus acts in the direction of self-preservation. But Orpha is also functioning in a hallucinatory and omnipotent manner as it lulls consciousness so as to deal with unbearable pain. With Orpha, any radical opposition between the life drive and the death drive, between creativity and destruction, between linking and unlinking, is put into question. Orpha is wise and connected to acts of survival in improbable circumstances, but it is ultimately a fragment; it is split off from other faculties. Orpha is formed when death is very near, but it acts as an organising life instinct.

Following up on the Ferenczian path, Michael Bálint (1937) proposed important ideas for thinking through the inheritors of ego instincts. He introduced the notion of 'primary love', or 'primary passive object love', and the characterological concepts 'ocnophilism' (referring to a tendency of relating to objects based on clinging on to them) and 'philobatism' (describing a relational tendency of crossing empty spaces and encountering obstacles). I see these contributions as attempts to ensure the inheritance of the ego-preservative drives and to tackle their disappearance from Freud's metapsychology.

Imagining Repetition: Ferenczi's Contribution

In 1920, Freud discovers a new kind of repetition which is not in service of the pleasure principle. When he solidifies this important discovery, because of its strong anchoring in the primacy of the death drive, he closes the path to exploring other kinds of repetition. Our imaginary on repetition became partly 'frozen' after the uncovering of its 'demoniac' aspect. In a succinct formulation, in 'Beyond the Pleasure Principle', Freud theorises two types of repetition. The first one is in service of the pleasure principle, and it proceeds by linking. It happens in the transference, in the psychoanalytic setting, and it leads to recollection. The second type of repetition is in service of the death drive, and it is an attempt to restore a previous state of things, an attempt to return to the inanimate by way of a total extinction of tension in psychic life. It is this second kind of 'demonic' repetition that represents the core discovery of the text 'Beyond the Pleasure Principle'.

The question I ask here is: what if there exists a track of repetition that does not directly serve the pleasure principle, nor does it bear its first and most important connection to the death drive? Can we come to conceive of a *reconstructive repetition*, in relation to the ego, aiming at eliminating residues of unworked-through traumas and at restoring a pre-traumatic state of the ego (or of the proto-ego)?

Let us start from a different notion, that of the 'affectionate current' in psychic life. In the early editions of *The Three Essays of the Theory of Sexuality*, Freud (1905) referred to the 'affectionate current' to designate the energies of the self-preservative drive and to the 'sensual current' to designate the libidinal energies in children. He also distinguished tenderness or affection [*Zärtlichkeit*] from sensuality [*Sinnlichkeit*]. Both the affectionate and the sensual current have as their first object the maternal breast. The relationship between the two currents is that of 'leaning on' (or anaclitic): when the baby is nursing, the sensual current leans on the affectionate current. The breast thus becomes the anaclitic object, or the object leaned upon [*Anlehnungsobjekt*]. In the last version that Freud proposed for his *Three Essays*, however, the affectionate current had lost its distinctiveness from the sensual current and took the more restrained and also negative form of inhibited sexual desire. In other words, it became sexual desire that cannot achieve full object love. In 1914, Freud had already formulated his ideas on primary narcissism. The theory of narcissism worked to efface the metapsychological autonomy of the self-preservative drive. What was once 'the affectionate current' was now depicted as a kind of narcissism.

While Freud spoke of 'the affectionate current' but failed to give it a destiny in his metapsychological texts, Sándor Ferenczi was the one to point out that self-preservative drives need reality from the very start. Even if we wish to speak of the life in the womb, there as well we find the reality of the functioning of the mother's body.

Ferenczi took a significant step in giving a relational form to the affectionate current, proposing a crucial dichotomy between the language of passion and the language of tenderness. Children experience as traumatic the interruption of the register of the language of tenderness, which is about gentle care and meeting basic needs, when they encounter the language of passion of the adults, in which repression and guilt are central. Is it the case that the language of tenderness holds the key to recapturing some of the spirit of the ideas contained in Freud's underdeveloped metapsychological ideas on the affectionate current in psychic life? And, an even more challenging question, how do we clinically have access to the moment at which the language of passion intrudes into the language of tenderness?

As mentioned above, Freud already marked a strong discovery of his own in 'Beyond the Pleasure Principle', which already pluralises our understanding of repetition. But this should not inhibit us from looking for other tracks of repetition, which are more capable of being in a productive connection with the observations we make in our contemporary clinical material.

Ferenczi's *reliving* maintains its specificities, even though at first instance it might appear to come close to the idea of traumatic repetition formulated by Freud in 'Beyond the Pleasure Principle'. It is worthy of being investigated as *a different track of repetition, grounded in a different metapsychology*. In brief, we can say that Ferenczi gave a whole different meaning to the series repetition/remembering/reliving. Freud contrasted remembering with repeating and had sharply distinguished between insight (memory or recollection) and experience (repetition or regression). Ferenczi saw repetition, and particularly regression or experiential reliving, as one of the tracks of remembering. Reliving is the way to gain access to the child within the adult, or what Ferenczi (1931a, p. 126) speaks of in terms of 'child analysis in the analysis of adults'.

This kind of reliving is grounded in a different proposition on temporality than any of Freud's ideas about *Nachträglichkeit*. As John Fletcher (2013) shows in his book *Freud and the Scene of Trauma*, Freud had remained, in his entire work, haunted by an idea of the authenticity of the scene of trauma. It is fair to say that while this haunting receives important elaboration in the passage from the first theory of trauma (the seduction theory) to the second theory of trauma, which gives status to fantasy (and thus seems to be pushing aside the disquieting questions about the authenticity of the original traumatic event), the theme of authenticity remains an important undercurrent even in writings that come long after the second theory. Laplanche and Pontalis (1968) rightfully point to the fact that the supposed 'abandoned' theory of seduction, which is one of the commonplaces of thought among commentators of Freud, actually contains many points that Freud preserved or returned to at later moments. Arguing along the same lines, Nicholas Rand and Maria Torok (1997) have stressed the oscillations between giving primacy to fantasy and giving primacy to the external event in Freud's thought. All these complicated returns are played out concepts such as the screen memory, the primal fantasy [*Urphantasie*], originary fantasy [*ursprünglich Phantasie*] and transference. That Freud was never able to set aside his questions about the authenticity of the traumatic event is only a statement of his untiring commitment to the understanding of human suffering. There is no easy resolution to the matter of the authenticity of the originary traumatic event; but there are more or less useful theoretical-clinical elaborations on this matter.

Ferenczi explored new solutions to the problem of authenticity and articulated the importance of achieving a sense of authenticity in relation to the traumatic experience as part and parcel of the very process of healing. In consonance with the role that the third recognising presence has in the Ferenczian theory of trauma, the psychoanalyst becomes an agent of recognition, allowing the emergence of a sense of authenticity that the patient never had access to before.

In Ferenczi's theory, memory operates both through the ego and through the id, constituting two different regimes or tracks of memory, defined in their difference by their object-relatedness (Stanton, 1991, p. 84). In the regime of id memories, we find 'bodily sensations', referring to primal life and death trends [*zugen*]. When these are elaborated retrospectively by the ego, they are lived as emotions. In the regime of ego memories, we encounter 'projected sensations', referring to the environment and to external occurrences. These tend to produce effects of objectivity, and they are experienced as verifiable consciously. The crux of the matter is how these regimes of memory interact and whether the emotionality of the bodily sensations and the objectivity effects of the projected sensations come to be connected. We can argue that Ferenczian reliving aims at a composition between id memories and ego memories.

Ferenczian repetition has its own track because it involves the memory register that has been constituted around bodily sensations. It is thus very far from mere remembering (which, in Freudian terms, would be the 'colder' activity of the conscious part of the ego, or the passing of marks from the unconscious part of the ego to the conscious part of the ego). Ferenczian repetition is also oriented towards the clearing up of traumatic residues – we could call it *reconstructive repetition* (occurring in dreams and even in certain forms of regression or in enactments in the psychoanalytic frame). Finally, it stands in a curious relation to the idea of restoring a previous state of things, which in Freud is interpreted as restoring the inanimate state, where tension is absent. What is being restored in a Ferenczian paradigm, in my view, is *a pre-traumatic state of the ego or of the proto-ego*. This form of reconstruction, therefore, passes through the self-preservative instincts or the ego instincts. In other words, we need the ego instincts in order to understand how this form of repetition works. It can only secondarily be said to operate in service of the pleasure principle, because it is more strongly marked by the operation of the self-preservative instincts. To conclude, without the implication of the register of memory of the id, the re-attunement between emotionality and rationality, which became split from each other at the time of the trauma, cannot be achieved.

A Ferenczian Rereading of Nachträglichkeit

Let us take some space for a comment on Freud's important system of ideas around *Nachträglichkeit*. Strachey's translation is that of 'deferred action'. As this translation suggests a linear temporality, some more felicitous translations have been attempted by Thomä and Cheshire (1991) as 'retrospective attribution' and by Laplanche (1998) as 'afterwardsness'. *Nachträglichkeit* refers to a temporal logic that governs the psychic world, and where we have a system of 'scenes', a kind of psychic scenography emerging through the effects of *interaction* between different moments in time (Birksted-Breen, 2003; Dahl, 2010; Faimberg, 2007; Fletcher, 2013). In short, the traumatic consequences of the first scene are only released in the form of a (hysterical) symptom as a result of the retrospective action of the second scene, which has the power to reactivate or revitalise the memory traces of the first scene. As Freud explains when he discusses the case of Katharina, the memory of the first scene persists in a defensively isolated state, in a kind of limbo, or 'in storage'. It is somewhat like a foreign body, constituted by way of the intensity of the excitation experienced at the time. The second scene reactivates it by way of connections and homologies. There is thus no exclusive power of the initial mnemonic trace, but the power emanates precisely from the interaction between the different moments. The effect of afterwardsness depends on the articulation of the various scenes, and crucially it includes processes of defence and repression.

John Fletcher (2013) takes us through some very interesting tensions that pass through the Freudian system of notions around the *Nachträglichkeit.* Crucially, in my reading, he points to Freud's insistence of the centrality of the first scene (which he will then trace back to an originary seduction scene). He refers to the other scenes as 'auxiliaries'. This statement on auxiliaries is counterintuitively accompanied by the assertion that there is a kind of infantile sexual indifference or apathy in relation to the first scene of abuse. The first scene only gains its status through the occurrence of the subsequent ones. Thus, memory comes to be lived as a contemporary event. In simpler terms, without the second moment, there would have been no trauma in the first moment. This thesis on infantile sexual indifference or apathy is very difficult to defend. It installs a certain sense of equality among mnemic traces that is also implausible. The idea of a very fragile ego, still unable to handle certain types of stimulation and easily broken by overstimulation, is not accounted for in this articulation.

It is here that the Ferenczian metapsychology of fragmented psyches can lead to useful questionings. The young fragile ego is neither apathetic nor indifferent; on the contrary, it is very sensitive to the moments when adults cease to address it in what Ferenczi referred to as 'the language of tenderness' and start to address it in the incomprehensible and overburdening (at the time) 'language of passion', which is specific to a register of sexuality that is unliveable by the child but at the cost of the fragmentation of the ego. While Freud would say that there was no trauma as such in the first moment, with Ferenczi we come to understand how the selection between the mnemic traces is made, so that not all memories have the potential of the subsequent contribution to the complicated palimpsest of different scenes and temporalities that can constitute a 'trauma'. In brief, it is the stimulation of the child via the language of passion that results in the 'pool' of scenes that the psyche can then weave, by composing different temporalities, into a trauma.

In what follows, I would like to discuss the quality of the relation between the different scenes/elements that come to constitute a trauma. Fletcher (2013) suggests that in the construction of his idea of 'screen memories' Freud is primarily guided by a metonymical logic. This means that 'the displacement from experience to screen takes place [...] between two adjacent elements within a simultaneous ensemble' (Fletcher, 2013, p. 116). Fletcher goes on to argue that Freud oscillates between this metonymic interpretation of memory (where there is a substitution of insignificant for significant parts within a large whole) and a metaphoric interpretation (where the elements are put in a relation of similitude or analogy). It is crucial to note that in his *Nouveaux fondements pour la psychanalyse*, Jean Laplanche (1987) proposed a use of the couple metaphor/metonymy that is crucial in making sense of the functioning of the life drive and the death drive, respectively.

According to Laplanche, the death drive and the life drive are two aspects of the sexual drive. The life sexual drive corresponds to a total and totalising object; it is linked (which in a Freudian sense, in Laplanche's account, means that it is maintained as more or less coherent and not split into pieces) by a relation to an object in view of or in process of an act of totalisation (Laplanche, 1987, p. 144). This means that the life drive is more inclined to metaphorical than to metonymical displacements. This is the case because precisely the kind of structures that present a certain totality, a certain internal articulation, are susceptible to become the matter of analogies. It is this act of gesturing towards some sort of totality that makes an operation of analogy thinkable. The death drive seems to correspond more to metonymical operations because it is always achieving a partial object – in Kleinian terms, an object that is unstable, formless and in fragments. In this reasoning, it is of crucial importance that we can qualify a relation between different elements as metaphorical or metonymical.

This brings us to Sándor Ferenczi, to his conception of the symbol, and to his ideas on analogical thinking. Association – linking across levels of sensoriality and signification – brings an alteration of material structures and a reorganisation of the very fleshiness of the body. Ferenczi is in dissonance with the Saussurean division of the sign into two constituent parts, material signifier (the word) and conceptual signified (the thing referred to by the sound). For him, things mean in their immediate materiality. Meaning is not detached, abstracted and located elsewhere. Materiality is not merely a lower order that entraps us, while the higher order of semantic fullness remains a horizon that we aspire for. '[T]he symbol – a thing of flesh and blood', he writes in 1921. The word-presentation [*Wort-Vorstellung*] can only deceivingly be equated with the symbolic. A word is at best a fossil outside chains of associations that include different sensorial impressions and thing-presentations [*Sach-Vorstellung*].

Although our space here does not allow a full reflection on a Ferenczian semiotics, it is crucial to mark the way Ferenczi differentiates 'unsubstantial allegory' from 'the symbol'. Not every analogy is symbolic in a psychoanalytic sense. The symbol emerges from a particular kind of *affectively charged non-arbitrariness*. How so? First, the symbol has a physiological basis; it 'expresses in some ways the whole body or its functions' (Ferenczi, 1921a, p. 355). Second, one of the two terms (things, ideas) of the analogy that can be considered symbolic is invested in consciousness with an inexplicable overcharge of affect. This surplus of affect is rooted in the unconscious identification with another thing (or idea) to which it actually belongs. When Ferenczi distinguishes between unsubstantial analogy and symbolic analogy, he contrasts the bi-dimensionality of the first with the three-dimensionality of the second. But what is the third dimension that he is referring to? I argue that the 'third dimension' is the analogical work of the mind/body of the analyst, linking the two series of elements that bear a homology (while having one of the series invested with inexplicable affect). The psychoanalyst thus works with symbols that are things 'of flesh and blood'.

The implications of seeing the symbol as an affectively charged non-arbitrariness are profound. I would here like to ponder on the idea of the non-arbitrary that emerges from Ferenczi's work and from his philosophical ideas on mimetism and analogy. Even language imitates the body and body parts in a complicated manner. This means that associations have a *necessary* aspect to them, and thus they also need to be very *precise*. Marion Oliner (2013) has recently helped us see that although there is a growing body of work in psychoanalytic theory on the 'irrepresentable', the 'non-represented' or 'non-represented mental states' (André Green, René Rousillion) we are still confronted with an unsettling clinical-empirical puzzle in the fact that there is often a very striking *accuracy* in the enactments and actualisations of the traumatic events, even when the memory of them remains inaccessible to consciousness. This is to say that the psychosoma is able to re-stage the traumatic events with a great level of precision.

It is this precision and minuteness of detail that leads us to believe that the crux of the matter is not that these marks were not presented in any way to the psyche or that they belong to the realm of the irrepresentable. Oliner (2013) uses 'non-represented' in inverted commas to draw our attention to the overuse of this term for situations in which what is actually missing are the associations between different modes of representation (or, we would say, between different modes of presentation in the psyche). The crux of the matter, rather, is another Ferenczian theme: that of the *splitting* of the psyche during a moment of excessive stimulation, when the psyche cannot convert the amount of free energy invading it into linked energy. In short, we can say that the reason why association is at times very difficult and painful across different sensorial modalities is because we are dealing with modes of presentation belonging to different split-off parts of the psyche, rather than because the traumatic event has not presented itself to the psyche in any way that produces a mark.

Returning to Freud, this brings a significant challenge to the thesis of the infantile sexual indifference. All the details that appear in the reliving of the traumatic scene must have made a sensorial inscription, which was retained in some way. The choice of elements in the traumatic scene and their relations are non-arbitrary. Also, non-traumatic memories compose details that needed to have had a personal significance at the time of their selection. Freud got disturbingly far from being able to account for why one *particular* scene (and not another one!) out of the countless moments of a child's life becomes the scene of trauma; and why some sensory elements and not others are tied into a non-traumatic memory.

The Ferenczian reading of *Nachträglichkeit* would entail, firstly, a psychoanalytically plausible version of a type of 'time-travel', where, via what Ferenczi calls memory of the id, or sensorial memory, we become able to 'touch' (here, I use 'touch' as a metaphor for multi-sensorial access, not just the strictly tactile one – it may be acoustic, olfactive, kinetic etc.) another time. Secondly, a Ferenczian *Nachträglichkeit* also involves a third presence in the structure of the traumatic scene, which 'locks-in' the trauma via denial (or misrecognition of the nature or of the magnitude of the child's experience, whose world was broken by the intrusion of the language of passion of the adult). When, in a clinical setting, different sensorial modalities become linked with one another and the memory of the id becomes connected in stronger ways to the memory of the ego, what we achieve is *effects of authenticity* which are at the core of the process of healing. Originally, the trauma brought the splitting of sensorial modalities and of parts of the more or less developed ego, producing *effects of inauthenticity*. It is crucial to mark that the memory of the id is capable of some form of inscription. This means that both in the 'locking-in' of the trauma, and in its subsequent unpacking and working-through, the memory of the id has a leading role. The reliving of a different moment in time and the recuperation of the split-off parts of the ego unfolds *in the spirit of the marks inscribed via the memory of the id*. In other words, healing occurs guided by and in the spirit of the memory of the id. This is perhaps the most psychoanalytically plausible version of authenticity that we can arrive at.

A Ferenczian reading of Freud's 'Beyond the Pleasure Principle' leaves us in a stronger position and brings us closer to understanding what was lost with Freud's 1920 text. In Ferenczi's work, there is a consistent investment in exploring the inheritors of the ego-preservative drives through his ideas on trauma, on the 'Orpha' fragment of the psyche, on the symbolic, and on healing. With Ferenczi, we can come to imagine a creative repetition, linked to the operation of the ego-preservative drives. The Ferenczian *Nachträglichkeit* is somewhat narrower than the Freudian one as it acknowledges the precision of the traumatic marks, the subsequent precision of their re-enactment, and the more limited operation of the death drive in their organisation. Kerz-Rühling (1993) stressed the difficulties of a purely hermeneutic conception of *Nachträglichkeit.* The radical clinical implication of such a hermeneutic reading would be that analyst and analysand can construe close to anything together, free from any necessity of the actual suffering of the original event. I have argued here that they construe in the spirit of the memory of the id, while grounding themselves in the force of the ego-preservative drives.

What sustains the psychoanalytic process and what makes it possible to 'glue' back together the split-off and deadened parts of the traumatised self is precisely the work of the ego-preservative drives, the instincts for harmony and sharing that Ferenczi was referring to in his diary entry of 13 August 1932, cited above. Healing is also sustained by a curious fragment of the psyche, by 'Orpha', the organising life instinct, found in a limbo between the life drive and the death drive.

The Event of Survival

While Ferenczi insists that the adaptive potential 'response' of very young children to sexual or other passionate attacks is much greater than one would imagine, it is worth stressing that what is at stake is not necessarily an act of sexual abuse. Indeed, what is at stake is a *psychic transmission*. In 'On Shock', Ferenczi clarifies this point: 'Shock can be purely physical, purely moral, or both physical and moral. Physical shock is always moral also; moral shock may create a trauma without any physical accompaniment' (Ferenczi, 1932c, p. 254). As Jay Frankel (2015) has shown, the place of the aggressor here is occupied in most cases by a narcissistically compromised caregiver. The 'attack' therefore consists of parts of the caregiver's mind intruding into the child; appropriating aspects of the child's mind and using it for the caregiver's own purposes (Frankel, 2015); or inverting the parent-child relationship, so that it responds primarily to the caregiver's needs and not to those of the child (Frankel, 2015).

The first response to the attack is a state of traumatic paralysis, which is incompatible with any sort of psychic spontaneity or activity of psychic defence. The paralysis is not a fleeting state or a moment of adaptation. Instead, it is capable of changing the structural organisation of the psyche, and it generates a 'frozen fragment' of the psyche, which is silent, deadened and fully de-libidinised. This frozen fragment moves outside of time and any sense of unfolding. As Ferenczi describes:

> First, there is the entire paralysis of all spontaneity, including all thinking activity and, on the physical side, this may even be accompanied by a condition resembling shock or coma. Then there comes the formation of a new—displaced—situation of equilibrium. If we succeed in making contact with the patient even in these phases, we shall find that, when a child feels himself abandoned, he loses, as it were, all desire for life or, as we should have to say with Freud, he turns his aggressive impulses against himself. Sometimes this process goes so far that the patient begins to have the sensations of sinking and dying. He will turn deadly pale, or fall into a condition like fainting, or there may be a general increase in muscular tension, which may be carried to the point of opisthotonus.
>
> (Ferenczi, 1931a, pp. 137–138)

The absolute paralysis of motility in the moment of the attack includes the inhibition of perception and, with it, the inhibition of thinking (Ferenczi, 1931b, p. 240). The traumatic impressions that occur at the time of the attack cannot be recorded via the system of memory of the ego, because this would involve the presence of thinking, even if we are talking about processes of repression. These impressions are thus taken up by the psyche without any sort of resistance. While Ferenczi hesitates between suggesting that 'no memory traces of such impressions remain, even in the unconscious, and thus the causes of the trauma cannot be recalled from memory traces' (1931b) and describing instead the elements of the new system of memory of the id, I have shown that the precision of the traumatic re-enactments leads us to believe that some marks, in the first instance incompatible with thoughts, are presented to the psyche.

The fact that the traumatised subject survives, psychically and physically, the moments of traumatic paralysis is a highly improbable event, in terms of the state of the drives. In other words, it is a time that is so radically dominated by the operation of the death drive and so prone to un-linking that the 'event of survival' requires an explanation.

Alongside the 'frozen fragment' of the psyche that moves outside time, there are other psychic forces at play. Ferenczi speaks of a psychic dimension always latent in the soma and, interestingly enough, in all material substance. This manifests as a series of ontogenetic and phylogenetic inclinations (or 'motives'). Ferenczi discusses this primal substrate in the first pages of his *Clinical Diary*, pointing to a process when different organs or body parts produce effects of thinking and are able to perform surprisingly minute calculations that have as a result the preservation of life.

> Inorganic and organic matter exist in a highly organized energy association, so solidly organized that it is not affected even by strong disruptive stimuli, that is, it no longer registers any impulse to change it. Substances are so self-assured in their strength and solidity that ordinary outside events pass them by without eliciting any intervention or interest. But just as very powerful external forces are capable of exploding even very firmly consolidated substances, and can also cause atoms to explode, whereupon the need or desire for equilibrium naturally arises again, so it appears that in human beings, under certain conditions, it can happen that the (organic, perhaps also the inorganic) substance

> recovers its psychic quality, not utilized since primordial times. In other words the capacity to be impelled by motives [*Bewegtwerden durch Motive*], that is, the psyche, continues to exist potentially in substances as well. Though under normal conditions it remains inactive, under certain abnormal conditions it can be resurrected. Man is an organism equipped with specific organs for the performance of essential psychic functions (nervous, intellectual activities). In moments of great need, when the psychic system proves to be incapable of an adequate response, or when these specific organs or functions (nervous and psychic) have been violently destroyed, then the primordial psychic powers are aroused, and it will be these forces that will seek to overcome disruption. In such moments, when the psychic system fails, the organism begins to think.
>
> (Ferenczi, 1932a, pp. 5–6)

In the hour of the traumatic attack, the event of survival means maintaining a beating heart or getting air into the lungs, against all odds. All available psychic energy is concentrated on one task, an apparently simple one, but without which preserving life would be impossible. The heart, at this time, becomes a 'thinking' heart.

Unlike the Kleinian 'projection' of the unwanted aspects of the self, we encounter in Ferenczi's work a curious libidinal act that can be read more as a temporary re-location or ex-corporation of the ego, rather than a mere projection. In his text 'On the Analytic Construction of Mental Mechanism', Ferenczi (1930a, p. 222) will call this ex-corporation of the ego 'getting beside oneself'. This psychic act requires remarkable amounts of psychic energy. The ego leaves the body and observes from outside, usually from above, the scene of suffering going on beneath. (I discuss this state at length in the following chapter.)

This 'othering of the self' produces dissociation and a sense of exteriority from one's own experience, which remains available to the self after the event, in situations that mimic the scene of the trauma. Often, this state is associated with a particular kind of timelessness: the subject feels triumphant over time or feels like they have overcome time or 'killed' time altogether. The time resulting from 'being beside oneself' attacks the sense of unfolding of the more conscious and well-adapted parts of the ego.

Among the fragments of the psyche that result from the unbearable attack in the moment of the trauma, we find a curious fragment that Ferenczi names 'Orpha' – the feminine of Orpheus. Orpha is perhaps Ferenczi's most complicated and eventful fragment, a kind of structural effect of self-caring in the psyche. (The next chapter is dedicated to Orphic functioning.)

The Time of Reliving on the Couch: Neo-catharsis

If the psyche presents itself as a kind of mosaic of parts, some of which are alive and some of which are deadened (de-libidinised), then what does it mean to say that some form of reconstruction is possible, and what does such a reconstruction rest upon? In his *Clinical Diary,* Ferenczi makes an intriguing note: 'in a manner which to us appears mystical, the ego fragments remain linked to one another, however distorted and hidden this may be' (Ferenczi, 1932a, p. 176). To achieve a fresh start in thinking about psychic healing we are to think about this note as a metapsychological assumption, rather than a metaphorical statement. This is confirmed by the fact that the 'link' preserved between the split parts of the psyche also makes its apparition in dreams and dream-like images and states. Patients sometimes bring us dreams of a cut-off body part that is still attached by one thread to the body. In such dream imagery, what is represented is not only the severed organ/head but also the thread that connects it to the body.

If we take this proposition seriously, what emerges as a question is: where and how can this thread be found and in which way can it be used for psychic healing? In the consulting room, this question brings us to the crucial importance of reliving for approaching the trauma. The clinician will know that as a result of a traumatic shock, one part of the personality can 'die' (or, in other words, the libido can fully withdraw from a part of the personality), while the part that survives the trauma can wake up from the shock with a 'gap in memory' (or, to be more precise, with a gap in conscious memory, or the system of memory of the ego). The 'thread' that we are discussing passes through the system of memory of the id, which has an entirely different inscription mechanism from the system of memory of the ego. This does not mean that nothing was ever presented or preserved in the unconscious but that, to be able to access it, a reliving by way of regression is needed. Ferenczi noted that often in the second part of the analysis what the patient experiences is a 'collapse of the intellectual superstructure', accompanied by a 'breaking through of the fundamental situation, which after all is always primitive and strongly affective in character' (Ferenczi, 1931a, p. 140). This kind of regression will make possible a 'new beginning' – a term that Michael Bálint (1968) will later put at the centre of his propositions on 'benign regression' and 'the basic fault'. What is repeated in this event of reliving is the original conflict between the ego and the environment and the painful intrapsychic solutions found for this conflict, in search of a fresh outcome.

This is where the experience of the 'trance' becomes relevant. It is however not any kind of mystical trance but precisely 'neo-catharsis', an experience of reliving the inscriptions made in the memory of the id while arriving at some effects of reality, veracity and conscious memory, in the presence of the analyst:

> It was easy to utilize these symptoms as fresh aids to reconstruction—as physical memory symbols, so to speak. But there was this difference—this time, the reconstructed past had much more of a feeling of *reality and concreteness* about it than heretofore, approximated much more closely to an actual *recollection*, whereas till then the patients had spoken only of possibilities or, at most, of varying degrees of probability and had yearned in vain for memories. In certain cases these hysterical attacks actually assumed the character of *trances*, in which fragments of the past were relived and the physician was the only bridge left between the patients and reality. I was able to question them and received important information about dissociated parts of the personality.
>
> (Ferenczi, 1929a, p. 119)

One difficult question is the nature of the fundamental difference between re-enactments driven by the compulsion to repeat, and operating under the imperatives of the death drive, and this form of 'neo-catharsis'. In other words, what precisely makes it possible for us to say that the reliving of the traumatic experience occurred under 'new conditions' (and potentially with a new resolution)? Here, the picture painted in Ferenczi's work is a complicated one, but there are two recurring themes. One new condition is that of the constant elaboration by the analyst of their own 'professional hypocrisy' (1933), referring to the analytical posture that makes the patients repress their criticism directed to their analysts, just as they repressed their criticism of lack of love from the adults in their childhood. As he notes:

> We greet the patient with politeness when he enters our room, ask him to start with his associations and promise him faithfully that we will listen attentively to him, give our undivided interest to his well-being and to the work needed for it. In reality, however, it may happen that we can only with difficulty tolerate certain external or internal features of the patient, or perhaps we feel unpleasantly disturbed in some professional or personal affair by the analytic session. Here, too, I cannot see any other way out than to make the source of the disturbance in us fully conscious and to discuss it with the patient, admitting it perhaps not only as a possibility but as a fact.
>
> (Ferenczi, 1933, p. 158)

This sort of clinical sincerity makes it possible for the patient to experience the traumatic events of the past as thoughts or as objective memories and not only as hallucinatory reproduction.

The second way to reach a new condition is to aim towards horizontality in the analytic space. Because of the ubiquitous nature of phenomena of infantile obedience, there will certainly be little scope for any complete or enduring horizontality, but the analyst needs to invent new ways around and across submission. Ferenczi (1932a, p. 108) argues that

> [t]he most essential aspect of the altered repetition is the relinquishing of one own's rigid authority and the hostility hidden in it. The relief that is obtained thereby is then not transient and the convictions derived in this way are also more deeply rooted.

The analyst's complicated work is to engage in some form of dialogue with psychic fragments that are already entangled in violent temporal relations. The crux of the matter then is intervening in these fraught temporal relations or finding ways to use the 'odd' times of some of the psychic fragments for the progress of the analysis.[1] In several entries of the *Clinical Diary*, Ferenczi describes the experience of engaging the Orpha fragment of the psyche. On the couch, Orpha appears as a fragment of the psyche that sometimes instructs, directs or guides the analyst with great precision as to what to do, how to speak, how to be silent, in order to allow the reliving of the traumatic sequence of events. In evoking the experience with one of his patients, Ferenczi writes:

> At her demand and insistence, I help her by asking simple questions that compel her to think. I must address her as if she were a patient in a mental hospital, using her childhood nicknames, and force her to admit to the reality of the facts, in spite of their painful nature. It is thought two halves have combined to form a whole soul. The emotions of the analyst combine with the ideas of the analysand, and the ideas of the analyst (representational images) with the emotions of the analysand; in this way the otherwise lifeless images become events, and the empty emotional tumult acquires an intellectual content.
>
> (Ferenczi, 1932a, p. 14)

> Proposal of a woman patient, O.S.L during the trance, simulate thinking by asking very simple questions, to revive tactfully yet energetically the 'ghost' which has been given up, as it were, and slowly to persuade the dead or split-off fragment that it is not dead after all. Simultaneously the patient must encounter enough compassion and sympathy that it seems worth his while to come back to life.
>
> (Ferenczi, 1932a, pp. 39–40)

In his piece 'The Two Extremes: Credulity and Scepticism', Ferenczi speaks of 'psychognosis' or 'gnosis' which he sees as 'the hope that it is possible, through an adequate profound relaxation, to gain access to a direct path to a past experience, which can be accepted without any other interpretation as being true' (Ferenczi, 1932b, p. 263). Here, the pre-traumatic time and the post-traumatic time touch. What we arrive at through 'psychognosis' is not direct access to the experience of how things truly were but an effect of authenticity and an effect of veracity. The post-traumatic state is, paradoxically, fuller in possibilities for enrichment and more radically relational than the pre-traumatic state.

Vignette: On Falling and Floating

Ella arrived in my consulting room shortly after an attempted suicide. A few weeks before, she had taken all her medication at once, a combination of antidepressants and sleeping pills. Her husband had found her and she was taken to the hospital in time, avoiding any permanent damage to her physical health. In the first session, she told me a lot about her dissatisfaction with her relationship, her feeling trapped in a couple with an older man with whom she fought often. She was able to talk directly about her suicide attempt, and she asked me for help. Her speech did not lack emotion and I found her expressive, but I also felt a heaviness and darkness at the core of what she was recounting. At times, it was as if a metallic sphere was slowly coming towards me.

The second session brought a surprise: Ella told me the same sequence of episodes she had evoked in the previous session, using the same words and the same voice inflections. It was an uncanny repetition, and as the minutes of the session passed, I felt the metallic sphere even heavier. In the second half of the session, I intervened and told her that I knew the story she was telling me already. I added that the story was familiar to me because she had told it to me in the previous session, but that I did not mind hearing it twice, or however many times she needed to tell it. She revealed that she had no recollection of having told me the same things in the previous session. She was occupied by chains of stories which she was telling herself and, at times, other people, but without shifting the words or the colour of her voice. For the first part of her analysis, I often felt like a recording device storing encrypted sequences which were hiding something dangerous.

After a few months, Ella moved to the 'dangerous place' in my presence and she told me her secret. When she was around four years of age, she was playing in the house of her mother and stepfather. In their house, one of the rooms was covered by a glass ceiling. Ella thought she saw a doll on the glass ceiling, to which she could get through a side entrance, and she went to get it. While crossing the ceiling, it collapsed with her. She fell with it on to a table, where her stepfather and his guests were seated, and glass shattered and spread everywhere. While she was screaming on the table, her mother came and spanked her and scolded her for having broken the ceiling, while the stepfather stood and watched, doing nothing. Ella had never forgotten what had happened; she had conscious knowledge of it, but a part of her psyche was in a pulverised state, just like the glass ceiling breaking into thousands of pieces. She was constantly falling and re-falling: her vocabulary around falls, drops, trips, tumbles and plummets was incredibly diverse. When she felt like she didn't want to go on with life, she experienced a blank and memory-less state where she would not take the pills but 'fall' into her box of pills. When she was experiencing uncontrolled emotions, she would tell me she was afraid of 're-falling' into one of the bad states. As a child, she was often left alone for long periods, taking care of herself and also of a brother a few years younger than herself, who had a neurological diagnosis. She was also ruthlessly beaten by both her mother and her stepfather. Given this extreme abandonment, I was often confronted with the sense of how improbable the event of her survival was: indeed, she had had to invent new organs to preserve her life in such circumstances. Self-caring was imperative, as she could not count on care by an other. But free-falling and total loss of control over the event of self-preservation was an equally active psychic possibility.

One of the important directions of our process was that of re-experiencing the fall and slowing it down. I worked with a vocabulary that 'transposed' what she brought in the session to another speed, always decelerating her movement: it was not free-falling and plunging, but floating, hovering, drifting slowly. This was also a form of addressing the traumatic progression that falling through the roof, as well as other episodes of abuse, had brought. Indeed, Ella was living across a-synchronic times to the point that these were tearing her apart, pulverising her sense of self and pulling her in different directions. A part of her was repeating in her mind a complaint and an accusation for mistreatment, like a lullaby or a soothing internal sound, without any sense about the thousands of times that she had repeated the exact same complaint to herself. Her repetitions were a self-caring sound. Another part of her was highly adapted: she completed her studies and obtained a position of considerable responsibility. Another part, perhaps the most dangerous one, was boundless and pulverised, like a cloud of particles without contour, existing outside time lived in its unfolding, experiencing herself as an effect of an inhuman, cruel and unstoppable acceleration. When this part of herself took over, she could 'fall' into the box of pills without having any recollection of engaging in a set of actions that happened in a sequence: taking out the pills from the bag, taking off the lid, counting the pills, swallowing the pills.

Several months after evoking the fall, Ella told me about a very conflictual situation with her husband, when she felt she had lost control. She suddenly remembered something else she wanted to show me and stood up from the couch, moving towards a chair in the consulting room where she had left her bag. While standing up, she paused and revealed that during the argument with her husband, she had picked up a vase and thrown it into a glass cabinet full of crystal glasses. The sliding doors of the glass cabinet were completely shattered. When telling me all this, she was making efforts to summon some feelings of shame for her 'losing control'. What I felt was that beneath a thin layer of self-reproach there was excitement and enjoyment. The way she told this story, as well, was 'derailing' from her usual grammar: there were pauses and seemingly un-related sequences. She was free-associating rather than voicing a background complaint. She was also standing up and looking at me, while I was following her from my chair. I intervened: in the past, when she had fallen through the glass roof, there was nothing she could control; now, when she broke the glass cabinet, she was standing and acting. Indeed, there had been some inversion between the horizontal and the vertical. For a moment, Ella could have a glimpse into her enjoyment in causing a derangement in the terrain of the pleasure in submitting and being subdued, which was dominating the relationship with her objects but also the relationship between different parts of her self.

A particular crossing of times was needed for our accessing and starting the analytic work with this 'alternative enjoyment', involving being active, doing, and causing. It was a combination of acting-out (breaking the glass cabinet) and acting-in (standing up and having part of her session while standing). Her standing up was akin to the state of 'trance' described by Ferenczi. She could relive part of her fall, but this time while standing, and while the analyst was acknowledging her psychic pulverisation and her suffering. The reliving in this case involved both the shattering of the glass cabinet (while in analysis) and the telling of this shattering (in the consulting room, while standing). This was the beginning of a long working-through of the scene of trauma. It took the form of the analytic pair engaging the violent temporal relations that the subject was living under. It was an instance of the time of reliving.

*

The clinical reimagining of *Nachträglichkeit* as implying a violent clash of times can produce important theoretical and clinical insights in psychoanalysis. Ultimately, there is a violent internal plurality of the times of the subject. Different psychic fragments 'live' inside a different time, creating an overall effect of a-synchrony. In other words, the times of some fragments attack, displace, or negate the times of other fragments.

On the Feminine Principle: On the Flip Side of the Drives

In what follows, I explore Sándor Ferenczi's ideas on 'the feminine principle', showing how it has clinical relevance today. Ferenczi articulates a vocabulary where terms such as conciliation, endurance of suffering, selflessness, appeasement, adaptation, renunciation, self-denial, and compromise percolate and are arranged in a surprising way, in a direct relation to his trauma theory. The feminine principle brings a rethinking of the reality principle and a re-evaluation of the duality of the drives. Ferenczi investigates the feminine principle while also being curious about unexplored forms of the life drive. The value of this 'life drive imaginary' emerges as something other than a naïve vitalism, a generic, optimistic image of the prevalence of life over death. In *The Clinical Diary,* Ferenczi (1932a) presents us with a particular modification to the sphere of the dualism death drive/life drive: he renames them the 'drive of self-assertion' and the 'drive of conciliation'. The 'selflessness' he evokes includes the 'selflessness' of organs: it emerges in relation to the scene of trauma and it ultimately describes a complex psychic state, which considers otherness and the relationship to the environment. The 'drive for conciliation' expresses the fact that in order to survive as any sort of individuality, one needs to practice a kind of politics of self-limitation. These ideas on 'the feminine principle' are tied to a revision of conceptions of genitality. Ferenczi invites us to democratise forms of erotism: he has in mind a clever combination of mechanisms of pleasure, and rich mixtures and transpositions of the erotic in psychic life.

Our point of departure is the observation that ever since Freud's 'Beyond the Pleasure Principle' (1920), clinical imaginaries have been dominated by the forms of the death drive. Here I ask questions about Ferenczi's orientation in relation to the 'alien body' of the death drive, in the context of his theory of psychic fragmentation. I argue that Ferenczi is productively ambiguous in relation to the death drive, and this productivity is manifested by introducing a series of disturbances in the two opposing series activity/masculinity/life drive and passivity/femininity/death drive, which produce conservative effects in psychoanalytic theory and in culture more broadly, and which write the feminine in the negative.

As I will show, Ferenczi does important work in pluralising our life drive imaginary. This comes with taking seriously the instances of radical plasticity of organs, psychic fragments, blood vessels or nerve fibres. In certain circumstances, organs and body parts are able to create new shapes or new configurations. Instead of insisting on either affirming or rejecting the duality of the drives, Ferenczi is more interested in the results of the fusion and the defusion of the drives or in how the death drive and the life drive 'compose' each other with more or less stable psychic results, often in relation to the forming of certain fragments of the psyche. Indeed, as Ferenczi writes in his 1924 book *Thalassa*:

> it seems more plausible to assume that a *complete* defusion of life and death instincts does not in general occur; that there are still 'germs of life' even in so called 'dead' matter, thus in inorganic matter; and accordingly, also, regressive tendencies to that higher degree of complexity from the disintegration of which they have originated.
>
> (Ferenczi, 1924, p. 94)

Later in the same text, he insists that: 'an absolute hegemony on the part either of life or of death is never attained' (Ferenczi, 1924, p. 94). Our challenge – both theoretically and clinically – is to gain insight into the complicated compositions of life drive and death drive. In other words, with Ferenczi, we can think about things that seem dead but prove not dead after all; things that seem alive but are stilled and unlinked in their core; things that become revivified; things that become dis-associated and unlinked; things that are bound both to the reality principle and to a particular kind of hallucinatory omnipotence associated to having survived the scene of trauma. The psychoanalytic process itself is construed in relation to this movement of revivifying, as it strives 'slowly to persuade the dead or split-off fragment that it is not dead after all' (Ferenczi, 1932a, pp. 39–40).

The Feminine Principle

To arrive at the construction of 'the feminine principle' as a matter of the drives, we can start with an exploration of how Ferenczi regards the feminine. My aim here is not to offer a full review of Ferenczi's writings on this theme, but to put together those elements that offer an interesting revision or dis-alignment to the Freudian view, or democratise our views, or disturb the unquestioned equivalence between femininity and passivity. It is undeniable that as a thinker and writer of his time, Ferenczi had in some of his writings suggested, for instance, a necessary link between accomplished femininity and motherhood or had treated the achieving of motherhood as a desirable outcome of the psychoanalytic process. But other texts escape this 'grid', and it is those that interest us here.

In an early text, the 1908 'The Effect on Women of Premature Ejaculation in Men' (published in the same year as Ferenczi's first encounter with Freud), we can register a significant contextualisation and historicisation of the condition of women-subjects in a patriarchal world. There are references to the 'selfishness' of men, and of physicians who are generally men, and who contribute to forming and maintaining a 'feminine ideal' (Ferenczi, 1908a, p. 291). This 'feminine ideal' actually brings a repudiation of active feminine sexuality and the relegation of the 'right' to sexual libido and orgasms to men alone. Women themselves adopt (or, should we say, are forced to adopt) this ideal. As Ferenczi writes, according to this ideal, women 'cannot admit or manifest sexual desire, but at most are allowed passively to tolerate it, with the result that, when libidinous tendencies manifest themselves in women, they are stamped as morbid or sinful' (Ferenczi, 1908a, p. 292). In a lucid analysis of the projection of patriarchal morals on women's lives, Ferenczi links forms of suffering such as anxiety neurosis, hysteria, or obsessional illness to the operation of the feminine ideal. While he does not use the word 'patriarchy', he does speak to and of patriarchy as an articulation of an oppressive system of social and moral laws. He also talks about the imposed 'sexual martyrdom of the female sex', which under conditions of patriarchy is faced with 'the appalling dilemma of choosing between complete satisfaction and self-respect' (Ferenczi, 1908a, p. 292).

Over two decades later, in *The Clinical Diary*, in an entry of 26 July 1932, we witness an important re-orientation in relation to feminine sexuality:

> Perhaps it was too hasty to represent feminine sexuality as beginning with the clitoris, with a shift of this zone much later to the vagina. It is even doubtful whether any organ at all can be thought of as 'undiscovered' by the psyche.
>
> (Ferenczi, 1932a, p. 174)

This is a striking re-democratisation of organs and their activity across the sexes. If the penis is discovered early by the boy-child, the vagina must also be discoverable and discovered by the psyche. My reading here is that we have an instance of Ferenczi writing female sexuality in an active register, thus taking steps towards what Lisa Baraitser has called 'de-gendering passivity and activity' (2023, p. 916).

Perhaps unsurprisingly, Ferenczi endorses 'psychobisexuality', according to which anatomical and psychosexual traces of the originally bisexual disposition are preserved and, under certain conditions, become dominant in an individual's psychic life (Ferenczi, 1908b, p. 21). 'Ambisexuality' thus refers to 'the child's psychical capacity for bestowing his erotism, originally objectless, on either the male or the female sex, or on both' (Ferenczi, 1912, p. 184, fn). Since Ferenczi is of the view that the psychological sexual traits in each individual are mixed, although in unequal proportions, sexual relations with one's own sex constitute only in some instances a 'disorder', while in many instances they are an expression of 'the normal life' of the soul (Ferenczi, 1911, p. 299). This constellation of statements, dispositions, orientations, and theoretical sketches make for an antipatriarchal and perhaps even a feminist view of female sexuality.

Against this backdrop, and towards the end of his life in an entry of *The Clinical Diary* on 4 August 1932, Ferenczi formulates an open critique of Freud for his 'androphile orientation' in theory and clinical practice:

> The ease with which Freud sacrifices the interests of women in favor of male patients is striking. This is consistent with the unilaterally androphile orientation of his theory of sexuality. In this he was followed by almost all of his pupils, myself not excluded. My theory of genitality may have many good points, yet in its mode of presentation and its historical reconstruction it clings too closely to the words of the master; a new edition would mean complete rewriting.
>
> (Ferenczi, 1932a, p. 187)

Ferenczi died before he could produce this exciting rewriting of his theory of genitality, which would have contained a critique of the androphile leaning of Freudian theory and also perhaps some positive manifestation of his own gynephilic orientation, which I believe he came to see as a necessary form of reparation for the tendency of the psychoanalytic field to sacrifice the interests of women. Ferenczi thought that, in comparison to the male, the female is, 'at least organically speaking [...] a more *finely differentiated being*, that is, one adapted to more complex situations' (1924, pp. 103–104). While such a view is not without its dangers of reproducing binaries, it is against this backdrop of a gynephilic disposition that Ferenczi will articulate the metapsychological construct he will call 'the feminine principle'.

Democratising Passivity

To make sense of 'the feminine principle', we need to address the question of passivity, teasing out the numerous and confusing ways this term is mobilised in psychoanalysis. Freud himself did not help us in clarifying these confusions. In other words, to stand any chance of creating a positive disturbance in the series femininity/passivity, we need to unpack some of the different meanings of passivity. I note here a sequence of stimulating questions that Lisa Baraitser has articulated in an effort to internally qualify and differentiate passivity:

> We might then ask, what is at stake now when we reconsider the conjunction femininity/passivity or masculinity/passivity? Is passivity really gendered? Do we need a concept of passivity to understand sexual difference? Can we do without it? Or is there something productive, even, in thinking 'with' passivity rather than passing it like the hot potato of psychoanalytic theory, between men and women, between the auto-affective male European subject and its many 'others'? Who, after all, is afraid of passivity?
>
> (Baraitser, 2023, p. 915)

After several close readings of Ferenczi's notes and fragments, and of his *Clinical Diary*, I am inclined to think that he was not afraid of passivity, and that his own explorations in the realm of passivity are of relevance today. In a little-known fragment written in 1930 called 'Thoughts on "Pleasure in Passivity"', he writes about a kind of drive passivity which is at the heart of 'the feminine principle'. To better understand this drive passivity, we would need to first contrast it with other key forms of passivity which are predicated on a different relationship with pleasure/unpleasure.

When 'passivity' is closely associated with 'femininity', it is most often in conformity with Freud's phallocentric conception. The body metaphor here is that of the clitoris that stops growing, as it actually reveals itself to be a stunted penis, or a penis that could not come into its own fullness. This idea is key to Freud's 1924 text 'The Dissolution of the Oedipus Complex'. This type of passivity is of the post-castration sort, where the little girl has not recovered (and cannot recover) from the disappointment of not being a little boy. As Jacques André (2014) suggests, this is a grammar of passivity where 'wounded' and 'passive' are equivalent – or a passivity of 'why bother?', where the psychic atmosphere is one of deadly stillness, inertia, disengagement and dis-investment. As Hélène Deutsch has put it: 'the absence of spontaneous vaginal activity constitutes the physiologic background of feminine passivity' (1944, p. 233). It is this understanding of passivity as activity turned inside out and transformed into inertia through a post-castration tragedy that constitutes the object of feminist critiques of psychoanalysis and the Freudian understating of female sexuality.

Taking a further step, we can discern a second paradigm of passivity, where passivity is not just the negation of activity. Freud gives some hints of this in his 1896 text on 'Heredity and the Aetiology of the Neuroses', where he aims to clarify the distinction between hysteria and obsessional neurosis. The 'event' that he places at the origin of hysteria is an event of passivity, 'an experience submitted to with indifference or with a small degree of annoyance or fright' (Freud, 1896, p. 155). Jacques André (2014) has called this a 'stupefied passivity'. I read it as the passivity of the one paralysed by the primal scene or by the trauma scene, of the one looking in from the outside, of the spectator with their gaze arrested, while they are being overwhelmed by the excess of excitation and by the psychic transmissions they are receiving from the other and from the scene itself. Here the position of the 'woman' can be interchangeable with that of a 'child'. It is a kind of primary passivity, where the fragile being is injured by the passions of the adult.

Turning to Ferenczi, there is a very important transformation that we can follow in the 'optics' of the trauma scene. What is particular to the Ferenczian scenography of the scene of trauma is that the child is included in the trauma scene, not looking from the outside or looking in on a scene in which the adults are acting. The psychic position of the child also has in its repertoire an extraordinary range of autoplastic transformations: it breaks itself up into fragments or even atomises itself, becoming matter without form; it mimics the shape of the aggressor, moulding a psychic fragment into the form of the aggressor; it grows strange new organs, usually related to attempts to psychically survive, albeit in fragments. All this autoplastic repertoire complicates any idea of a 'stupefied passivity': it suggests that most forms of passivity are unstable, and beneath a psychic 'surface' there is a richness of active solutions, even if they involve psychic fragmentation. This constitutes a reconfiguration of both passivity and activity and an important step to de-gendering passivity. Autoplastic solutions are not a feminine path or feminine destiny: they are democratised across the field of traumatisation, which includes all subjects.

Our last step here takes us to a third paradigm of passivity which for me is strongly related to Ferenczi's work and to his notes on 'the feminine principle', on 'pleasure in passivity', on 'pleasure in self-sacrifice', on 'altruistic pleasure' and on 'the pleasure of adaptation'. I discuss this series of constructs under the caption of 'drive passivity' to mark their connection with the operation of the drives. As we can see here, pleasure makes an important return in this set of terms. The crux of the matter is how can we make sense of pleasure in passivity that is not pathologically masochistic – and of forms of self-destruction and fragmentation that are not a pure manifestation of the death drive but instead constitute forms of fusion of the death drive and life drive. As Ferenczi writes in a short note of 1931: 'each adaptation is a partial death, a surrender of one part of the personality' (1931c, p. 243). I would like our accent here to be on 'partial' rather than on 'death'. The psychic atmosphere we are interested in is one where the arrival at a new ingenious composition of fragments is associated with a distinct form of pleasure. Let us further investigate this psychic atmosphere.

The Drive for Conciliation: Passivity and Oblique Stillness

Pluralising our imaginary of the life drive comes from taking seriously the instances of radical plasticity of organs and psychic fragments. Organs and body parts are able to reshape themselves or create new configurations. In Ferenczi's *Thalassa*, the immersion in the sphere of the life drive takes the form of an investigation of a variety of 'protective' formations that the psycho-soma can create. For instance, he looks at various ad hoc protective bladders, vesicles, pustulae filled with fluid, or 'places of abode', usually developed under the strain of the traumatic attack. Such protective creations are directly implicated in psychic survival at the time of catastrophe. There is a complex analogy at play here:

> the supposition that the amniotic fluid represents a sea 'introjected', as it were, into the womb of the mother – a sea in which, as the embryologist

> R. Hertwig says, 'the delicate and easily injured embryo swims and executes movements like a fish in water'.
>
> (Ferenczi, 1924, p. 11)

Ferenczi (1932a) constructs a whole new series of terms, which are both clinically and politically interesting: cooperation, conciliation, endurance of suffering, selflessness, appeasement, adaptation to renunciation, self-denial, compromise. In one entry of *The Clinical Diary,* he experiments with a particular modification to the sphere of the dualism death drive/life drive. He renames them the 'drive of self-assertion' and the 'drive of conciliation'. The 'selflessness' he evokes, including the 'selflessness' of organs, emerges in relation to the scene of trauma. The 'drive for conciliation' appears as the basis for the reality principle. To survive as any sort of individuality means to practice a kind of politics of self-limitation. Ferenczi names this 'the feminine principle' (1924).

The work of the drive of conciliation brings a slowness of reaction, or even a temporary non-reactivity, a stillness, or a 'passibility' [*passibilité* in French] that Dominique Scarfone (2019) and Lisa Baraitser (2023) discuss, drawing on Lyotard's notes (1988). Passibility is a quality of passivity linked to suffering or sensation. It marks a capacity to endure suffering or feeling – and an openness to being affected.

This state resonates with what Cornelius Castoriadis (1987) terms 'the shock of what is' (*Anstoß*) which is not a case of the environment causing a determinate outcome in the subject or the living being but a setting in motion of 'the formative (imaging/imagining, presenting and relating) capacities of the living being' (Castoriadis, 1989). It is thus a sort of creative and consequential collision with the environment. Literally, *Anstoß* is a 'stimulus' or a 'push'. The challenge is not to explain how the living being (or the subject) is determined by the environment but to explain how the living being's self-determination is *affected* by the environment. In other words, taking seriously 'the shock of what is' means that we take seriously the fact that we have a relationship with the world that lies beyond our representations. It is, however, an encounter that sets in motion the process of representation, which affects representations without determining them. Ultimately, this shock marks the capacity of the self for being affected.

In *Thalassa,* there is a moment when Ferenczi imagines the great catastrophe, the drying up of the oceans and marine creatures being forced to grow limbs and develop lungs to adapt to life on land. As Jenny Willner (2023) argues, they are creatures who 'would have preferred not to conquer land' – their plasticity is not expansive or triumphant but restrained, self-limiting.

The state that Ferenczi associates with the work of the drive of conciliation is one that is non-retaliatory, although it does not lose its inclination or leaning out in relation to the other. But in order not to clash, or retaliate, or destroy the other, one needs to point away from the other. I would describe this as a posture of *oblique stillness while pointing away from*. This posture is not neutral. Adriana Cavarero (2016) speaks about the gestures, alignments and misalignments of all those in history who, through their work of care, are more visibly inclined towards others. What results is a hidden geometry of postural care. Cavarero looks at how Western philosophy has produced a core image of a subject who is vertical, straight and self-balanced and who holds himself upright in relation to every other subject: the autonomous 'I'. This 'formal uprightness' (Cavarero, 2016) is also a paradigm of relationality: it configures the way in which care, social roles, norms, deviance, and bodies will be grasped. What is weaved out of the story is the 'inclined I', the subject who is not straight or vertical, but oblique or tilted. To be interested in obliqueness, inclinations and leaning towards the outside is thus a form of feminist critique.

A Psychoanalysis of Organs

The psychic states I have captured so far are not, however, some kind of normative ideal. They belong to a 'clinical empiricism', as their development starts in the consulting room, in the transference. Ferenczi explores a 'psychoanalysis of organs' which takes seriously the organ as a site of anxiety and signification and investigates some fascinating semi-autonomous qualities of organs. He introduces ideas such as 'organ neurosis' (1926) and even more curious phenomena such as 'organ individuality' (1924, p. 82) or the 'cooperation of organs' (1924, p. 82). Organs appear to have a secret life: they are capable of different kinds of regressions, perversions, strangulations, condensations, displacements, and doublings which we usually attribute to the psychic stratum (Wilson, 2015).

We enter a clinical imagery of 'wise organs'. As Ferenczi states: 'when the psychic system fails, the organism begins to think' (1932a, p. 6). The accent here is on the productive and materialising force of hysteria: the lump in the throat of the hysteric patient is not merely a hallucination but part of a new 'grammar' of organs, a stirring up of the tissues of the throat, or of the contents of the stomach, or of the intestinal matter, which implies a capacity for condensation, displacement, repetition, or identification. This showcasing of the creativities of the hysterical symptom has important implications for how we can imagine the relationship between the psyche and the soma. In short, there is a 'horizontalising' gesture here, where the soma is just as capable of complex acts as the psyche.

In *Thalassa*, Ferenczi (1924, p. 82) talks about an internal qualitative differentiation in the sphere of the libido which can lead to an 'organ libido' or even an 'organ individuality'. As he writes:

> According to the 'theory of genitality', the cooperation of organs and of their component parts does not consist simply of the automatic adding together of useful workmen to give a sum total of performance. Each organ possesses a certain 'individuality'; in each and every organ there is repeated that conflict between ego- and libidinal interests which, too, we have encountered hitherto only in the analysis of *psychic individualities*.
>
> (Ferenczi, 1924, p. 83)

Ferenczi differentiates between the 'altruistic' functioning of organs and autoerotic or self-gratifying processes in the tissues. Organs are thus capable of cooperation, but this is not a guaranteed outcome; it takes struggle and a complicated negotiation between opposing forces. The 'selflessness' evoked, including the 'selflessness' of organs, emerges in relation to the scene of trauma.

On the Flip Side of the Drives

There has been some controversy over whether Ferenczi 'dropped' the duality of the drives and especially the death drive (Avello, 1998; Cabré, 2003; Dal Molin et al., 2023). This is justified to the extent that there are several moments when he defends the duality of the drives – and others when he retracts from the death drive, such as his note of August 1932, where he writes: 'Nothing but life-instinct/death [instinct] a mistake (pessimistic)'. Rather than pondering on whether Ferenczi was 'for' or 'against' the death drive, or whether there is a movement in his work away from the death drive and in the direction of the life drive, I follow Ferenczi's *circling* of the death drive construct, while creating his own constructs (such as 'the feminine principle') and while voicing some productive ambiguities in relation to the death drive which can energise contemporary debates. In resonance with Jakob Staberg (2023), we can treat the death drive as a 'foreign object', stirring up the psychoanalytic field. In what follows, I pay close attention to Ferenczi's productive ambiguities in relation to the death drive and to the consequences of these ambiguities. In particular, I look at how Ferenczi sometimes preserves, and other times disturbs, the opposing series activity/masculinity/life drive and passivity/femininity/death drive. We are thus percolating on the flip side of the drives, where at times we can see the death drive turning itself into the life drive – or where we can spot death within life and life within death.

A first productive ambiguity takes place in the polarity pleasure/unpleasure by the affirmation of the principle of unpleasure [*Unlustbejahung*] – the ability to suffer, to wait, to tolerate frustration – which goes alongside the affirmation of a new kind of masochism. In effect, it is a masochism that needs a new name and that deflects from any simple conversion of unpleasure back into pleasure, in favour of a more qualitatively differentiated formula: the abolishing of a part of the self in the service of a form of survival, which can be of the self (but note that it is already a transformed self) or of an other. Ferenczi writes in *The Clinical Diary* on 26 April 1932:

> in any case, a quite different solution remains open, which says that not all masochism originates in fear, but also that kindness and self-sacrifice exist as instincts in their own right and are perhaps a natural force, keeping selfish impulses in balance.
>
> (Ferenczi, 1932a, p. 91)

In an earlier note written in 1930, Ferenczi details the 'pleasure of adaptation', which I understand as the pleasure of arranging various (surviving) psychic fragments in a new constellation while also losing some other fragments:

> In the moment when one must cease to use the environment as material for one's own security and well-being [...], one accepts the role of sacrifice, so to speak, with sensual pleasure, i.e. the role of material for other, stronger, more self-asserting, more egoistic, forces.
>
> (1930b, p. 225)

This disposition of accepting one's being 'material for the other' is also important in understanding the maternal function, which involves 'toleration of parasitic beings, which develop a completely egoistic manner at the expense of the mother's own body' (Ferenczi, 1932a, p. 42). Another instance of accepting being 'material for the other' is the very position of the psychoanalyst, which Ferenczi pictures as a particular kind of plasticity and willingness to give a part of the self for the other to use.

Remaining on the flip side of the drives means that we refrain from simply 'feminising' the death drive or placing a sign of equivalence between 'the feminine principle' and 'the death drive'. The feminine principle is not the feminine or maternal transubstantiation of the death drive. In my reading, it is precisely a readiness to traverse cycles that lead from pleasure to unpleasure and back again. And it is the ability to persist at the limit where life can be extinguished, at the same time that dead fragments can be revivified.

To trace Ferenczi's ambiguity and productive disorientation in relation to the death drive, let us look at two different entries of *The Clinical Diary* which were written only two months apart from one another. On 23 February 1932, he writes: 'The drive for self-assertion may be seen as the basis for Freud's pleasure principle, the drive for conciliation as the basis for his reality principle' (1932a, p. 42). This sentence condenses Ferenczi's insights on the drive for conciliation. However, on 26 April 1932, we are met with a question that turns on its head the previously suggested serialisation self-assertion/death drive/pleasure principle and conciliation/life drive/reality principle: 'should the death instinct be posited as an instinct of kindness and self-sacrifice, something maternal-feminine in opposition to the masculine?' (1932a, p. 91). This alternative series conciliation/death drive/feminine/maternal/altruistic appears again in a condensed note where Ferenczi writes just: 'Death=feminine, mother' (1932a, p. 183) and in the striking title of a short text of 1931, 'Aphoristic Remarks on the Theme of being Dead—being a Woman'. It might thus appear that Ferenczi is coding the feminine principle as the death drive. I would dispute that, as it is a certain kind of 'death' that is at stake here: is it a partial death, a death of a part of the self that has an orientation towards survival, of the self and of the other. For Jakob Staberg (2023), the 'feminine principle functions as a capacity for life, bordering on death at the same time as it acknowledges life beyond the individual'. In other words, the feminine principle is a re-socialising of life and survival. Surviving on one's own is unwise and fruitless.

The feminine principle thus implies its own kind of afterwardsness or *Nachträglichkeit*, or a significant unfolding, based on a crossing of two distinct moments in time. In a first temporality, it might appear closer to the death drive, because it involves auto-plasticity: the destruction of a part (or several parts) of the self. In a second temporality, it is closer to the life drive, because it involves the rebuilding of the self out of detritus: a kind of re-constellation of fragments. I return here to a section of *Thalassa*, which can ground this reading:

> It may be that the 'altruism' therein expressed is merely the clever combination of rudimentary egoisms; but it is also entirely possible that the degree of complexity already attained acts upon the products of disintegration in the manner of a regression or at least contributes thereto, that organisms are not so eager to die but that they can and do rebuild themselves out of their own detritus – nay, utilize for this renewed development the *vis a tergo* which they received on the occasion of their partial destruction.
>
> (Ferenczi, 1924, p. 90)

This takes us to a fundamentally non-dualistic horizon, where no duality can be posited (or eternalised) and where there is a circular movement that constantly re-arranges the pairs activity/passivity, masculinity/femininity, life drive/death drive and egoistic/altruistic. This non-dualistic thinking is the ground for Ferenczi's sketch for a revised theory of sexuality.

Towards a Revised Theory of Sexuality

I have argued elsewhere (Soreanu, 2023) that in *Thalassa* (1924) Ferenczi makes a de-Oedipalising intervention. I am referring to Ferenczi's (1924) idea of *amphimixis of eroticisms*, a construction that can impact the way we think through different forms of relationality. His focus is not on component instincts, but on the outcome that they can lead to through their *encounter* while understanding that this will not be peaceful, harmonious, or conflict-free. It may be a clash. Ferenczi talks about the fusion of different eroticisms, containing different pleasurable and painful experiences, with different object relations and forms of displacement in a way that transcends any strictly *individual* horizon of reference. He names the fusion of eroticisms 'amphimixis' – a medical term that denotes the mingling of two substances, usually to create a third. In Greek, the prefix 'amphi-' means 'on two sides'. There is no unilinear, irreversible or progressive sexual development of the individual, but rather every act we might wish to analyse will be a mix of infantile, adult, oral, anal and genital components. This mix will be unique and irreducible to these components. Amphimixis refers to individuals, but also to their *relations*. As I see it, amphimixis is at the heart of a radical revision of sexual theory.

This non-dualistic and non-linear thinking constitutes a democratisation of forms of erotism. Ferenczi creatively de-centres the genital register; he displaces the primacy of the genital over the other component instincts. His language is 'horizontal', as he argues that:

> The genital would then no longer be the unique and incomparable magic wand which conjures erotisms from all the organs of the body; on the contrary genital amphimixis would merely be one particular instance out of the many in which such fusion of erotisms takes place.
>
> (Ferenczi, 1924, p. 12)

Genitality is read in *Thalassa* as a retrogression to the original striving of being immersed in the womb and its gratifications. But beyond the genital amphimixis, the psyche is capable of 'a clever combination of mechanisms of pleasure' (Ferenczi, 1924).

There is a pressing need for psychoanalysis to grapple with the ways in which it has written the feminine in the negative and has indeed repudiated femininity. An interesting route for addressing this repudiation is to experiment with a metapsychology constructed in the feminine, where the connection between the construct and biological sex is never straightforward but a 'machine' for producing relevant questions. Another equally important route is to de-gender and dis-associate the series of terms which have historically been gendered in a binary way with conservative effects: the masculine with its association to the life drive and to activity – the feminine with the death drive and passivity. I have discussed elsewhere (Soreanu, 2023) that Ferenczi shows an interest in intermediary forms in the field of sexuality, which are *neither/nor*, or are *both/and* if we consider the categories of feminine and masculine. The implications of this double move are wide-ranging, and can result in a revised theory of sexuality. My reading is that Ferenczi's 'feminine principle' is a new drive, composing the pleasure of adaptation with the pleasure of self-destruction. This new drive is relational, where the subject is inclined in relation to the other and to the environment, or in a position of oblique stillness while pointing away from the other.

Note

1 'Each 'adult', who 'takes care of himself' is split (is no single psychic unit). Apparent contradiction: Sense of reality is possible only on the basis of a 'fantasy' (=unreality) in which a part of the person is sequestrated and is regarded 'objectively' (externalized, projected); this, however, is only possible with the help of a partial suppression of emotions (repression?) – Analyses which are carried through on the level of reality never reach the depth of the processes of splitting. Yet each succeeding development depends on the way it occurs (on its vehemence), on the time factor, and on the conditions, of the original splitting (primal repression). Only in earliest childhood, or before the original splitting, was anyone 'one with himself'. Deep analysis must go back under the level of reality into pre-traumatic times and traumatic moments, but one cannot expect a proper resolution unless this time the resolution is different from the original one. Here intervention is necessary (regression and new beginning). Cf. the kindly understanding, the 'permission to give vent' and the encouraging calming reassurance ('Suggestions')' (Ferenczi, 1932d, pp. 270–271).

References

André, J. (2014). Femininity and passivity in the primal scene: The little death of Sardanapalus. In: J. Fletcher & N. Ray (eds), *Seductions and Enigmas: Laplanche, Theory, Culture*. London: Lawrence & Wishart.

Avello, J. J. (1998). Metapsychology in Ferenczi: Death instinct or death passion? *International Forum of Psychoanalysis*, 7: 229–234.

Bálint, M. (1937). Early developmental states of the ego: Primary object love. In: *Primary Love and Psychoanalytic Technique* (pp. 90–108). London: Karnac, 1994.

Bálint, M. (1968). *The Basic Fault. Therapeutic Aspects of Regression*. London: Tavistock.

Baraitser, L. (2023). Passivity and gender: Psychical inertia and maternal stillness. *International Journal of Psychoanalysis*, 104(5): 912–926.

Birksted-Breen, D. (2003). Time and the après-coup. *International Journal of Psychoanalysis*, 84: 1501–1515.

Cabré, L. J. M. (2009). Ferenczi's 'feminine principle': A feminine version of the death drive. *American Imago*, 66(4): 411–418.

Castoriadis, C. (1987). *The ImaginaryIinstitution of Society*. Cambridge: Polity Press.

Castoriadis, C. (1989). The state of the subject today. *Thesis Eleven*, 24: 5–43.

Cavarero, A. (2016). *Inclinations: A Critique of Rectitude* (transl. by A. Minervini & A. Sitze). Stanford, CA: Stanford University Press.

Dahl, G. (2010). The two time vectors of *Nachträglichkeit* in the development of ego organization: Significance of the concept for the symbolization of nameless traumas and anxieties. *International Journal of Psychoanalysis*, 91: 727–744.

Dal Molin, E. C., Coelho Junior, N. E., & Cromberg, R. U. (2023). Ferenczi's variations on the death drive. *American Journal of Psychoanalysis*, 83(2): 231–249.

De Masi, F. (2015). Is the concept of the death drive still useful in the clinical field? *International Journal of Psychoanalysis*, 96: 445–458.

Deutsch, H. (1944). *The Psychology of Women: A Psychoanalytic Interpretation.* New York, NY: Grune and Stratton.

Faimberg, H. (2007). A plea for a broader concept of *Nachträglichkeit. Psychoanalytic Quarterly*, 76: 1221–1240.

Ferenczi, S. (1908a). The effect on women of premature ejaculation in men. In: *Final Contributions to the Problems and Methods of Psycho-analysis* (transl. by E. Mosbacher, pp. 291–295). London: Karnac, 1994.

Ferenczi, S. (1908b). The analytic interpretation and treatment of psychosexual impotence, in: *First Contributions to Psycho-analysis* (transl. by E. Jones, pp. 11–34). London: Karnac, 1994.

Ferenczi, S. (1909). Introjection and transference. In: *First Contributions to Psycho-analysis* (transl. by E. Jones, pp. 35–93). London: Karnac, 1994.

Ferenczi, S. (1911). The nosology of male homosexuality (homoerotism). In: *First Contributions to Psycho-analysis* (transl. by E. Jones, pp. 296–318). London: Karnac, 1994.

Ferenczi, S. (1912). On the part played by homosexuality in the pathogenesis of paranoia. In: *First Contributions to Psycho-Analysis* (transl. by E. Jones, pp. 154–184). London: Karnac, 1994.

Ferenczi, S. (1924). *Thalassa. A Theory of Genitality* (transl. by H. A. Bunker). London & New York, NY: Karnac, 1989.

Ferenczi, S. (1926). Organ neuroses and their treatment. In: *Final Contributions to the Problems and Methods of Psycho-Analysis* (transl. by E. Mosbacher, pp. 22–28). London: Karnac, 1994.

Ferenczi, S. (1929a). The principle of relaxation and neocatharsis. In: *Final Contributions to the Problems and Methods of Psycho-analysis* (transl. by E. Mosbacher, pp. 108–125). London: Karnac, 1994.

Ferenczi, S. (1929b). The unwelcome child and his death instinct. In: *Final Contributions to the Problems and Methods of Psycho-analysis* (transl. by E. Mosbacher, pp. 102–107). London: Karnac, 1994.

Ferenczi, S. (1930a). On the analytic construction of mental mechanism. In: *Final Contributions to the Problems and Methods of Psycho-Analysis* (transl. by E. Mosbacher, p. 222). London: Karnac, 1994.

Ferenczi, S. (1930b). Thoughts on 'pleasure in passivity'. In: *Final Contributions to the Problems and Methods of Psycho-analysis* (transl. by E. Mosbacher, pp. 224–227). London: Karnac, 1994.

Ferenczi, S. (1931a). Child-analysis in the analysis of adults. In: *Final Contributions to the Problems and Methods of Psycho-analysis* (transl. by E. Mosbacher, pp. 126–142). London: Karnac, 1994.

Ferenczi, S. (1931b). On the revision of the interpretation of dreams. In: *Final Contributions to the Problems and Methods of Psycho-analysis* (transl. by E. Mosbacher, pp. 238–243). London: Karnac, 1994.

Ferenczi, S. (1931c). Aphoristic remarks on the theme of being dead – being a woman. In: *Final Contributions to the Problems and Methods of Psycho-analysis* (transl. by E. Mosbacher, pp. 243–244). London: Karnac, 1994.

Ferenczi, S. (1932a). *The Clinical Diary of Sándor Ferenczi*, ed. by J. Dupont (transl. by M. Bálint & N. Z. Jackson). Cambridge, MA: Harvard University Press, 1995.
Ferenczi, S. (1932b). The two extremes: Credulity and scepticism. In: *Final Contributions to the Problems and Methods of Psycho-analysis* (transl. by E. Mosbacher, pp. 263–264). London: Karnac, 1994.
Ferenczi, S. (1932c). On shock. In: *Final Contributions to the Problems and Methods of Psycho-analysis* (transl. by E. Mosbacher, E., pp. 253–254). London: Karnac,1994.
Ferenczi, S. (1932d). Integration and splitting. In: *Final Contributions to the Problems and Methods of Psycho-analysis* (transl. by E. Mosbacher, pp. 270–271). London: Karnac, 1994.
Ferenczi, S. (1933). The confusion of tongues between adults and the child. In: *Final Contributions to the Problems and Methods of Psycho-analysis* (transl. by E. Mosbacher, pp. 156–167). London: Karnac, 1994.
Fletcher, J. (2013). *Freud and the Scene of Trauma*. New York, NY: Fordham University Press.
Frank, C. (2015). On the reception of the concept of the death drive in Germany: Expressing and resisting an 'evil principle'? *International Journal of Psychoanalysis*, 96: 425–444.
Frankel, J. (2015) The persistent sense of being bad: The moral dimension of the identification with the aggressor. In: A. Harris & S. Kuchuck (eds), *The Legacy of Sándor Ferenczi: From Ghost to Ancestor* (pp. 204–222). London & New York, NY: Routledge.
Freud, S. (1896). Heredity and the aetiology of the neuroses. In: *Standard Edition* (Vol. 3, pp. 141–156). London: Hogarth Press.
Freud, S. (1905). Three essays on the theory of sexuality. In: *Standard Edition* (Vol. 7, pp. 125–243). London: Hogarth Press.
Freud, S. (1911). Formulations on the two principles of mental functioning. In: *Standard Edition* (Vol. 12, pp. 213–226). London: Hogarth Press.
Freud, S. (1914). On narcissism: An introduction. In: *Standard Edition* (Vol. 14, pp. 67–102). London: Hogarth Press.
Freud, S. (1920). Beyond the pleasure principle. In: *Standard Edition* (Vol. 18, pp. 3–64). London: Hogarth Press.
Grubrich-Simitis, I. (1993). *Back to Freud's Texts*. New Haven: Yale UP.
Kerz-Rühling, I. (1993). Nachträglichkeit. *Psyche*, 47(10): 911–933.
Laplanche, J. (1987). *Nouveaux fondements pour la psychanalyse*. Paris: PUF.
Laplanche, J. (1998). *Notes sur l'après-coup* [Paper presented at the Conference on psychoanalytical intracultural and intercultural dialogue. International Psychoanalytical Association, Paris, 27–29 July].
Laplanche, J., & Pontalis, J.-B. (1968). Fantasy and the origins of sexuality. *International Journal of Psychoanalysis*, 49: 1–18.
Lyotard, J.–F. (1988). *L'inhumain. Causeries sur le temps*. Paris: Galilée.
May, U. (2015). The third step in the drive theory. On the genesis of Beyond the pleasure principle. *Psychoanalysis and History*, 17(2): 205–272.
Oliner, M. (2013). 'Non-represented' mental states. In: H. B. Levine, G. S. Reed, & D. Scarfone (eds), *Unrepresented States and the Construction of Meaning: Clinical and Theoretical Contributions* (pp. 152–171). London: Karnac.
Rand, N., & Torok, M. (1997). *Questions for Freud: The Secret History of Psychoanalysis*. Cambridge, MA: Harvard University Press.
Scarfone, D. (2019). The feminine, the analyst and the child theorist. *International Journal of Psychoanalysis*, 100(3): 567–575.

Soreanu, R. (2023). Toward a psychoanalysis of organs: A note on Ferenczi's contribution to the theory of sexuality. *Imago Budapest*, 12(3): 43–53.

Staberg, J. (2023). Complicated dialogue: Ferenczi (re-)reading Beyond the pleasure principle. *Imago Budapest*, 12(3): 30–42.

Staberg, J. (2024). Ferenczi thinking beyond the pleasure principle. In: H. Westerink, J. Willner, & P. Van Haute (eds), *Towards the Limits of Freudian Thinking: Critical Edition and Readings of Beyond the Pleasure Principle* (pp. 257–283). Leuven: Leuven University Press.

Stanton, M. (1991). *Sándor Ferenczi: Reconsidering Active Intervention*. London: Free Association Books.

Thomä, H., & Cheshire, N. (1991). Freud's *Nachträglichkeit* and Strachey's 'deferred action': Trauma, constructions and the direction of causality. *International Journal of Psychoanalysis*, 18(3): 407–427.

Van Haute, P., & Westerink, H. (2024). From repetition and drive monism to binding and conflict: Re-reading Freud's beyond the pleasure principle. In P. Van Haute, H. Westerink, & J. Willner (Eds.), *Towards the Limits of Freudian Thinking: Critical Edition and Readings of Beyond the Pleasure Principle* (pp. 165–196). Leuven University Press.

Westerink, H., & Van Haute, Ph. (2022). *Verleiding, drift en herhaling. Freuds metafysica van het trauma*. Amsterdam: Boom.

Willner, J. (2023). Catastrophes and genitality: Ferenczi's *Thalassa* and the politics of bioanalysis. In: R. Soreanu, J. Staberg, & J. Willner (eds), *Ferenczi Dialogues: On Trauma and Catastrophe* (pp. 91–130). Leuven: Leuven University Press.

Wilson, E. A. (2015). *Gut Feminism*. Durham, NC: Duke University Press.

Young-Bruehl, E. (2011). The trauma of lost love in psychoanalysis. In: S. Akhtar & M. K. O'Neil (eds), *On Freud's 'Beyond the Pleasure Principle'* (pp. 250–264). London: Karnac.

Chapter 3

The Times of Orpha

Orpha, a New Psychic Agency

Images of creatures watching a scene from above – such as angels, gods or other superhuman entities – are very familiar in painting. In a detail of the mural by Rodolfo Morales, four floating heads are watching over a collective scene – a procession – where people are walking into a fantastical fold made up by other giant human figures. They are perhaps joining their ancestors. It is often the case that analysands who have gone through great suffering refer to the scene of trauma by relying on images such as: 'I was looking down at myself from the ceiling'; or 'it seems that a part of me was watching over all this'; or 'it's strange that when I remember this it's as if I was seeing it from above'; or 'I floated up to the ceiling, I was not down there'; or 'I could see myself down there but I was also above it all, up high, at a distance'. What psychic formation can account for this possibility of distancing, of floating above the scene, of watching over the unfolding as if it was a performance executed somewhere 'below' the point of perspective? What kind of optics to the scene of trauma allows this split between a part of the self that is undergoing the aggression or being overwhelmed, and a part of the self that is watching all this from above? In the following pages, I engage with the conditions of possibility for this type of splitting and for this psychic formation. I do so in dialogue with Sándor Ferenczi's ideas on the 'Orpha fragment' of the psyche, which appear in some of his late work, especially in the *Clinical Diary*.

My interpretation is that Orpha is a fourth 'agency' of the psyche. This offers an important revision to Freudian metapsychology. Orpha can be considered alongside the id, ego and superego: it is a psychic system, not just a mechanism of defence, as I will show. The splitting processes related to the formation of Orpha are forms of *narcissistic splitting*. Under the strength

DOI: 10.4324/9781032715926-4

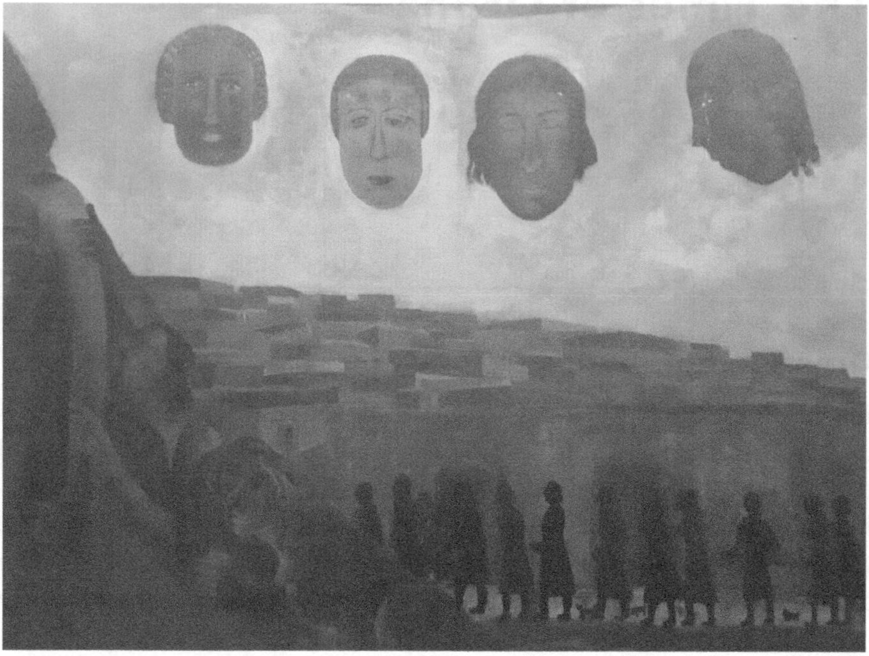

Figure 3.1 'Los que llegan con sus recuerdos e se van con sus flores' by Rodolfo Morales (1994), mural.

Photograph by the Author.

of the traumatic attack, the psyche is forced to devise new ways to care for itself, and at times the only way to do so is by fragmenting itself into *parts that care* and *parts to be cared for*. We are thus speaking about a tragic narcissism of fragments, where the self does not take itself for an object, like in the Freudian story of narcissism, but the self treats one of its parts as an 'other' and takes *it* as an object. A narcissism of fragments comes with very particular forms of denial. It also comes with what Ferenczi calls 'autosymbolism' (Ferenczi, 1930a, p. 221) which can be understood as an effort to find an expression for a psychic state of being in fragments by focusing a great part of the libido on body parts or organs. These organs become a corporeal symbolisation of the psychic splits. The body can make a meaningful arrangement, can swell up, or resorb, or relocate one of its parts, so as to make an inscription about the state of psychic fragmentation.

In the *Clinical Diary*, we come across a new vocabulary which allows us to imagine the psychic life of the Orpha fragment of the psyche. Among the terms of this new vocabulary, I note: 'guardian angel' (Ferenczi, 1932a, pp. 8–10 & pp. 102–106); 'ancient substitute (to thinking)'; 'substitute mother' (Ferenczi, 1932a, pp. 102–106); 'dissociation of fragments and organs'; 'explosion'; 'destruction of psychic associations'; 'anarchy of organs (where reciprocal cooperation is compromised)' (Ferenczi, 1932a, pp. 68–70). It is important to examine this vocabulary and to see where it can take us in terms of making sense of *psychic phenomena of self-caring*. In this context, self-caring refers to little-understood psychic positions such as the ones I evoked above, where a part of self is watching over the other part of the self that is undergoing the suffering. It is equally important to look at how Ferenczi arrived at his formulation of 'Orpha', as this was a particular form of co-creation with one of his patients, Elizabeth Severn (Rachman, 2017; Rudnytsky, 2017, 2021).

Ferenczi's 'pre-Orphic' vocabulary is important here as well. I will explore ideas such as 'getting beside oneself'; 'traumatic progression'; 'autotomy'; 'neo-formations'; 'teleplastia'; the 'wise baby'; and 'reconstruction'. All these represent a constellation of Orphic terms which I unpack by drawing on clinical vignettes and literary fragments that evoke Orphic psychic atmospheres.

In analysing the plurality of splits that constitute 'Orphic formations', I also discuss the psychic temporalities of Orpha. I ask: how are Orphic times experienced in the psyche, and also how do they appear in the transference, in the consulting room? I reference a particular kind of 'eternal present' as the main temporality of Orpha, but I also look at other 'strange' times that are associated with Orphic functioning. The Orphic eternal present is linked to the event of having survived an overwhelming attack by the other, of staying alive in conditions where survival would have been an improbable event. As I will show, Orpha is characterised by particular forms of omnipotence, of a psychic triumphalism that posits (in a hallucinatory manner) that, because the subject has survived *this* violent psychic event, they can survive any other attack or challenge, thus being invulnerable or unbreakable. This sense of invulnerability goes alongside an eternal present and a series of moments that are not linked up in a sequence. In this eternal present the subject seemingly iterates: 'I can do everything' or 'I can do anything'. I will discuss below the qualities and implications of this psychic time and look at how this temporality makes its presence felt in the consulting room.

The fact that Orpha is the feminine of Orpheus and is written as a 'feminine' psychic agency is a puzzling thing. I believe it is not to be seen as 'gendering' metapsychology, with conservative and binarising effects. Ferenczi writes his theory of the drives from the position of someone animated by the question: 'what can the feminine do?' and 'what can we do with the feminine?' He has a desire to repair some of the Freudian 'androphile' orientations, which he criticises (1932a, p. 187). I see the fact that Orpha is written in the feminine as part of a 'gynephilic' orientation of Ferenczi. This means primarily a sensitivity to societal hypocrisy in relation to feminine sexuality, which is usually written in the negative and associated with passivity, serving a moralising 'feminine ideal' (Ferenczi, 1908).

Furthermore, as we are reminded by Peter Rudnytsky (2017) and Arnold Rachman (2017), Orpha starts from some observations made by analysand Elizabeth Severn, who had gone through multiple sexual traumas as a girl-child, and had experienced the split in which one part of the psyche is watching over and caring for another part of the psyche while the latter is in agony. It is Severn who named this split-off fragment in the feminine, and Ferenczi preserved its being named in the feminine. While Orpha's singular 'voice' as psychic fragment has been discussed by a number of contemporary authors (Hristeva, 2013, 2019; Smith, 1999), and I have previously written about it as well (Soreanu, 2018, 2023), we need to further understand how to relate to Orpha in the consulting room. That is what I propose below.

I draw on clinical vignettes from my consulting room, but also on literary fragments, which are used to enhance the clinical understanding of the psychic states I am capturing. I here create an 'alliance' with writer Amélie Nothomb, who in her fictional work grows a kind of internal ear, listening to the various voices of psychic fragmentation. The fragments speak, suffer, or are in dialogue with one another. It is as if we are able to hear the psychic scenes and discern the elements that make up these scenes. Entering a 'transcript' of psychic fragments, we get to hear entire parts of the psyche growing up too fast, or lagging behind, or stepping outside time, or attacking other times of the psyche, or eternalising the present, or reliving a moment of the traumatic past.

Getting beside Oneself and Seeing the Self as an Other

It is in his consulting room that Ferenczi records a curious libidinal and topical act: a temporary re-location or ex-corporation of the ego, a radical form of splitting that re-positions the two resulting parts of the ego at a distance from one another. In his text 'On the Analytic Construction of Mental Mechanism', Ferenczi will call this ex-corporation of the ego 'getting beside oneself' (1930b, p. 222). This psychic act requires tremendous psychic energy. Although this fragment is associated to a temporary state in the scene of the trauma, it is profoundly linked with the structuring of the Orpha fragment of the psyche. It generates a kind of psychic 'trail' that the psyche can later repeat or reconstitute in situations of abuse or strain:

> Another process requiring topical representation is characterized in the phrase 'to get beside oneself'. The ego leaves the body, partly or wholly, usually through the head, and observes from outside, usually from above, the subsequent fate of the body, especially its suffering. (Images somewhat like this: bursting out through the head and observing the dead, impotently frustrated body, from the ceiling of the room; less frequently: carrying one's own head under one's arm with a connecting thread like the umbilical cord between the expelled ego components and the body.)
>
> (Ferenczi, 1930b, p. 222)

Many clinicians working with traumatised patients have noted the peculiar fantasy of exiting the body, of observing oneself from the ceiling, as if the self were an other. This 'othering of the self' produces an important dissociation, a sense of exteriority from their own experience. This psychic position of exteriority to the self is available to the subject in subsequent situations that mimic the scene of the trauma. The psychic fragment 'observing from the ceiling' marks what I call a 'pre-Orpha function'. It develops after a moment of traumatic paralysis, where the subject is made 'still' by the force of the aggression coming from the other. This paralysis is experienced as a near-death, as a cessation of all thought and feeling. We can say it precedes the coagulation of the Orpha fragment of the psyche, which, as we will see, comes in the shape of a 'guardian angel' – a true, stable and fully shaped dissociation, capable of watching over the abused child, abandoned by all external helpers and subjected to the overwhelming force of the aggressor.

The psychic imagery that accompanies the formation of this psychic position is very striking. The subject does not only 'find' themselves looking from the outside at their own suffering but often has a sense of a physical journey to the new ex-corporated state. The movement can be that of leaving the body through the head. Another possible movement can be an image of 'losing one's head' and carrying it under one's arm. What is crucial here is the representation of the dissociation of faculties. Seeing and thinking (standing for objective perception) are relocated elsewhere, while the rest of the body is left in agony on the ground (standing for affect).

In his *Clinical Diary*, Ferenczi makes a series of interesting observations on this distinctive topical catastrophe of the scene of trauma. He clarifies the alterations to the sense of time that come with the act of 'getting beside oneself'. He points to a non-human or trans-human imagery that accompanies the ex-corporation. The subject no longer feels reduced to spatial and temporal constraints, acquiring a sense of a radical plasticity: they can be condensed, enlarged, or even change states of aggregation.

> If I am to believe what my patients report about similar states, this 'being gone' is not necessarily a state of 'non-being', but rather one of 'not-being-here'. As for the 'where', one hears things like: they are far away in the universe; they are flying at a colossal speed among the stars; they feel so thin that they pass without hindrance through the densest substances; where they are, there is no time; past, present and future are simultaneous for them; in a word, they feel they have overcome time and space. Seen from this gigantically wide perspective, the significance of one's own suffering vanishes, indeed there develops a gratifying insight into the necessity for the individual to endure suffering, when opposed and combatant natural forces meet in one's own person.
>
> (Ferenczi, 1932a, p. 32)

What we can discern here is a state of traumatic omnipotence and a particular kind of *timelessness*, where a part of the subject feels triumphant over time or feels like they have overcome time or 'killed' time altogether. Another way of thinking about it in terms of temporal relations is to consider a *bifurcated time of the self*, a disjunct and *self-multiplying present*, based on defiance in relation to spatial boundaries. Both the suffering part of the ego, lying on the floor in agony, and the ex-corporated part of the ego, which has hallucinated a perspective 'from the ceiling', live in their own *eternal present*. The former is a present of eternal suffering, while the latter is a present of eternal triumph over suffering and of fleeing from it to a place where all suffering has been abolished.

There is also a particular kind of alienation that derives from different parts of the psyche being in their own different present times. We have seen, already, that Ferenczi's ideas on psychic fragmentation imply a violent internal plurality of the times of the subject, where the different psychic fragments, each 'living' inside a different time, create an overall effect of *asynchrony*. The times of some fragments seem to attack, displace or negate the times of other fragments. Here, the time resulting from 'being beside oneself' attacks the sense of unfolding in the more conscious parts of the ego, or, in other words, it attacks a reliable sense of 'I am here'.

Traumatic Progression and De-Synchronising Parts of the Self

A great deal has been said in psychoanalysis about processes of regression, including by Ferenczi himself. Other members of the Budapest School of Psychoanalysis (such as Michael Balint) have left an important mark on seeing regression as more than just a pathological occurrence in the clinic. They insist that some forms of regression work in service of the psychoanalytic treatment, allowing previously unrepresented psychic states to become available for linking and symbolisation. Alongside his work on regression, Ferenczi illuminates a psychic process that is the psychic antithesis of regression: traumatic progression.

When subjected to an overwhelming psychic transmission or an attack, the child can go through an instantaneous maturation and develop the emotions of an adult. This accelerated coming of age is often accompanied by being able to perform roles more easily associated with motherhood or fatherhood than with childhood. The playful, spontaneous, gradual appropriation of the world stops, while the traumatised child migrates to a place of 'carer' for the narcissistically compromised adults around him, for other children, or even for parts of the self, as we will see further. Another facet of this precocity refers to sexual roles. It is worth noting that it is a *fragment* of the psyche that goes through what Ferenczi calls 'traumatic progression' or 'precocious maturity' and not the entire personality (Ferenczi, 1933, p. 165). A traumatic bifurcation takes place that produces both a markedly paternal/maternal fragment and other fragments that are still 'childful' in their needing the presence of the register of tenderness, of gentle care and gradual learning, in order to mature.

Traumatic progression extends to the sphere of the intellect: the traumatised child will be capable of surprisingly wise utterings, sometimes to the delight of the adults around them, who will gratify and encourage faculties that are in fact results of traumatic dissociation. As Ferenczi (1933, p. 165) poetically puts it: 'It is natural to compare this with the precocious maturity of the fruit that was injured by a bird or insect'. Ultimately, Ferenczi regards the intellect as born out of suffering.

The splitting that leads to the birth of intellect is recorded in the unconscious in the form of dreams where a 'wise baby' enters the scene, speaking in the voice and with the contents of an adult conversation. Babies in the cradle or very young children are present in these dreams, and they are able to talk or write fluently, they find solutions to complicated puzzles, they offer intelligent advice and guidance to adults, or they offer scientific explanations. Ferenczi (1923, pp. 349–350) records this type of dream in his short 1923 piece, 'The Dream of the "Clever Baby"', which I reproduce here:

> Not too seldom patients narrate to one dreams in which the newly born, quite young children, or babies in the cradle, appear, who are able to talk or write fluently, treat one to deep sayings, carry on intelligent conversations, deliver harangues, give learned explanations, and so on. I imagine that behind such dream-contents something typical is hidden. The superficial layer of dream-interpretation in many cases points to an ironical view of psychoanalysis, which, as is well known, attributes far more psychical value and permanent effect to the experiences of early childhood than people in general care to admit. The ironic exaggeration of the intelligence of children, therefore, expresses a doubt as to analytical communications on this subject. But as similar appearances in fairy tales, myths, and traditional religious history very often occur, and in the painter's art are also effectively represented (see the Debate of the young Mary with the Scribes), I believe that here the irony serves only as a medium for deeper and graver memories of their own childhood.

> Therefore the wish to become learned and to excel over 'the great' in wisdom and knowledge is only a reversal of the contrary situation of the child. One part of the dreams of this content observed by me is illustrated by the pithy observation of the ne'er-do- well, when he said, 'If I had only understood how to make better use of the position of the baby.' Lastly, we should not forget that the young child is familiar with much knowledge, as a matter of fact, that later becomes buried by the force of repression.
>
> (Ferenczi, 1923, pp. 349–350)

The 'wise baby' became an important psychoanalytic construction for Ferenczi, through which he was able to better discern the effects of the particular arrangement of the trauma scene on his patients. This dream plays an important role in understanding precocious maturity, a traumatic kind of maturity, or a sudden split between faculties, between reason and emotion, where the intellect comes to function autonomously and disconnected from both emotion and the body.

The wise baby reasserts the general situation of asymmetry in the psyche, where there is an interplay between a psychic position coded as all-powerful and a psychic position coded as all-vulnerable. This uneven distribution of power is relevant whether we are dealing with a scene of aggression or with a scene of care. The wise baby can be seen as an attempt at altering the all-vulnerable position through an unusual psychic solution: by acquiring some hyper-faculties.

In terms of temporal relations, the wise baby can be understood as a *radical de-synchronising* of parts of the self and their times. While one part is propelled into adulthood in an accelerated fashion – evoking fairy tales where we are told that the hero grows as much in one day as others would in seven days – another part is left behind and remains an 'eternal child', unable to mature and needing constant care. The precocious voice of the child might often be more manifest, but what it covers up is precisely this other 'arrested' child that cannot grow.

The Boy Who Sings

> *Kat and her analyst are on the train together. Kat has to get off the train, and at that point she sees that the analyst is holding on her lap a wise Spanish boy who sings. The boy is visibly very intelligent, and he*

can also sing beautifully. Kat looks from the platform inside the train and feels some longing and sadness in relation to the boy held in the analyst's lap.

The dream of the wise baby has appeared many times and taken many forms in my work with patients. Staying with the dream images of wise babies and allowing them to percolate has often led to fruitful work. Each 'wise baby' is singular, and the dream images contain clues related to the particularity of psychic fragmentation linked to the image. In the dream I recorded here, the analysand places a boy version of the wise baby in the analyst's lap. Further associations with the dream allowed Kat to recall that as a child she had an 'imaginary friend', a boy who was very wise and gave her guidance about how to carry herself in public and how to act in challenging circumstances. Both the memory of the imaginary friend and the dream image of the singing Spanish wise boy allowed Kat to elaborate on how femininity was repudiated in her family, how a series of violent intergenerational transmissions inscribed the feminine as an 'impossible' psychic position, while absent male roles were often idealised. The images also allowed us to get closer to her desire for both spontaneity and study (the boy in the dream could sing *and* think at the same time). In this dream, there is also a certain deviation from the 'wise baby' dreams that Ferenczi discusses: there, the wise baby is the one who is doing the caring, often performing superhuman tasks in the horizon of care. In Kat's dream, the wise baby is placed in the analyst's lap, temporarily allowing himself to be cared for, while Kat is watching with longing. This arrangement of the dream scene allowed Kat to connect with her desire to be cared for. Despite not sharing a mother tongue (the wise boy is Spanish, and so is Kat, while the analyst is not Spanish), the boy of the dream manages to communicate by singing beautifully. He is different, yet legible.

On the Death of Childhood

[...] I understand that, quite simply, you hardly love me at all, you love me so little that it doesn't even occur to you to hide your mad passion for this baby in any way. The truth is, Maman, that if there is only one virtue you are lacking, it is tact.

> *In that moment Diane stopped being a child. She did not become an adolescent or an adult: she was five years old. She was transformed into a disenchanted creature who was obsessed with not foundering in the abyss that this situation had created inside her.*
>
> *Maman, I have tried to understand your jealousy, and the only thanks I get is this abyss you have opened before me, into which you have fallen, and it even looks like you'd have me fall into it, too. But you won't get away with it, Maman, I refuse to become like you, and I can tell you, without even having fallen in there, just sensing the call of that abyss, it hurts so badly I could scream, it is like a void closing around me. Maman, I understand your suffering but what I don't understand is why you care so little for me, in fact you are not trying to share your hurt with me, you simply don't care if I suffer, you don't see it, it's the least of your worries, and that's the worst thing of all.*
>
> *She acted as if everything were fine. She had to. Diane kissed Célia as warmly as she could, and no one noticed the death of her childhood.*
>
> (Nothomb, 2017, p. 47)

This excerpt of Amélie Nothomb's novel *Strike Your Heart* captures a moment of traumatic progression when child-Diane realises the mother's lack of love for her, which goes alongside her registering the mother's love-charge for Diane's newborn sister, Célia. Diane had previously formed a successful defence against the realisation of the absence of love when, in the past, the mother gave birth to a boy-child. Diane had 'theorised' that while her mother can love little boys, she cannot love little girls, and this is the reason why she cannot love her. Upon the birth of her sister, this 'theory' was refuted, with catastrophic effects. Diane could now see that the mother could love little girls too, but she had just been unable to love Diane. It is a psychic transmission around the unavailability of love that here constitutes the traumatic event. This resonates with Ferenczi's (1929) discussion on the 'unwelcome child' and the 'dropped child': the fact that a child is treated as an unwelcome guest to the family, and not received with love, means that their 'positive life impulses and motives for his sub-sequence existence' (1929, p. 106) are not stimulated, and the child is thus abandoned in the domain of the death drive. Ferenczi considered that the infant is 'much closer to individual non-being' (1929, p. 105), that is, to the death drive; as such '[s]lipping back into this non-being might therefore come much more easily to children' (ibid).

Following the catastrophic discovery of being unwelcome and unloved, Diane matures in an instant; she becomes 'wise', distant, disenchanted, pessimistic, and also a cold 'judge' of her mother's character. Capturing a similar process, Ferenczi noted that unwelcome children often acquire traits such as 'moral and philosophical pessimism, scepticism and mistrust' (1929, p. 104). Diane coldly addresses her mother in fantasy: 'The truth is, Maman, that if there is only one virtue you are lacking, it is tact'. We can discern here the words and the tone of an adult. And we register the 'death' of Diane's childhood, which means the traumatic renunciation of the expectation of being cared for by an other. Betrayed and traumatically wounded, Diane both seemingly rejects the identification with her mother – 'I refuse to become like you' – and in effect identifies with the aggressor. She hides her psychic devastation, and in a controlled manner becomes capable of displaying love that she doesn't feel: 'She acted as if everything were fine. She had to. Diane kissed Célia as warmly as she could, and no one noticed the death of her childhood'. In this scene of psychic overexertion, Diane is split into fragments. Her faculties of observation are traumatically enhanced, but her affects are stilled, frozen, and so is her capacity for spontaneous play. In a moment, she had to become a carer and a self-carer; and so as to survive, she will need to live with the 'abyss' opened up in her psyche by having been 'dropped'.

Autotomy and the Repudiation of the Past

There are two kinds of responses of the ego to the trauma, according to Ferenczi. The first one, corresponding to a highly developed sense of reality, he terms 'alloplastic adaptation' which means that the ego is able to alter the environment, the world outside, in such a way that self-destruction and self-reconstruction are not necessary and the ego maintains its equilibrium (Ferenczi, 1930a, p. 221). The second one he names 'autoplastic adaptation' (ibid), which means that the ego does not have the capacity to mould the external world, or loses this capacity, and proceeds to operate on itself.

Perhaps the most tragic form of autoplastic adaptation is autotomia, where the ego seemingly cuts off, dis-attaches and leaves behind a part of itself. It is here that Ferenczi relies on the image of the animal shedding a body part that has been wounded. Let us think of lizards cutting off their tail. In 'Psycho-analytical Observations on Tic', Ferenczi writes:

> Here I will touch on the analogy of the third kind of tic, i.e. the motor discharge ('turning against one's own person', Freud), with a method of reaction that occurs in certain lower animals, which possess the capacity for 'Autotomia'. If a part of their body is painfully stimulated they let the part concerned 'fall' in the true sense of the word by severing it from the rest of their body by the help of certain specialized muscular actions; others (like certain worms) even fall into several small pieces (they 'burst asunder', as it were, from fury). Even the biting off of a painful limb is said to occur.
>
> (Ferenczi, 1920, p. 160)

In one of the entries of the *Clinical Diary*, Ferenczi (1932a, p. 179) brings another vignette on animal behaviour, where the adaptation to the anticipation of unbearable pain and complete submission is suicide:

> As an analogy I refer to a reliable account of an Indian friend, a hunter. He saw how a falcon attacked a little bird; as it approached, the little bird started to tremble and, after a few seconds of trembling, flew straight into the falcon's open beak and was swallowed up. The anticipation of certain death appears to be such torment that by comparison actual death is a relief.
>
> (Ferenczi, 1932a, p. 179)

Ferenczi derives crucial metapsychological reflections from these images. In the first one, on autotomia, we see 'an archaic prototype of the components of the masochistic instinct' (Ferenczi, 1920, p. 161). In the second one, we see the limits of passivity, and a certain primacy given to activity, in that an active death is preferred to the anticipation of complete surrender to the aggressor. In a fragment on 'Trauma and Anxiety', Ferenczi (1931c, p. 249) strengthens the same idea: '*[s]elf-destruction* as *releasing some anxiety* is preferred to silent toleration'. It appears that the conscious system is easiest to break apart, responsible as it is for the integration of mental images into a unit. Ultimately, splitting is an act that is more readily available to the psyche than we are used to consider. Autotomy refers to a kind of splitting in which a part of the psyche becomes permanently unavailable to any form of linking.

In terms of temporality, autotomia is a particular kind of repudiation of the past, where any chain of causality or meaningful sequential arrangement between different moments in time is denied. It is as if the subject is saying: 'nothing happened *then* and therefore there are no effects on the *now*'. The deadened part of the psyche is seemingly left behind, but it is very difficult to imagine that anything in the psyche is ever successfully 'lost'. This effect of severing the dead part is obtained by a radical de-investment, an unlinking. It is thus more accurate to imagine that the psyche now contains a deadened, unlinked and unsymbolisable part, rather than that the part has been truly 'left behind'. In the *Clinical Diary*, Ferenczi refers to this part of the psyche as 'unsymbolisable id'.

On Neo-formations

Psychic splitting is often associated with destruction, unlinking, and the forces of the death drive. Ferenczi observes how self-fragmentation and splitting are at times bound up with the creation of new organs and new capacities – or, as he calls them, 'neo-formations' (Ferenczi, 1926a). In his 1926 essay on 'The Problem of Acceptance of Unpleasant Ideas', he discusses how certain kinds of self-destruction lead to an enlarged recognition of the surrounding world and lead closer to the formation of objective judgement. Here Ferenczi cites Sabina Spielrein's (1912) paper on destruction as a 'cause of being', which is in itself notable, given the lack of acknowledgement of her ideas at the time. Those ideas seem, as Adrienne Harris (2015) comments, to have been absorbed rather than referenced, turning Spielrein into a ghost rather than an ancestor. Resonating with Spielrein, Ferenczi argues that a partial destruction of the ego is tolerated but only with the purpose of constructing a stronger and more resilient ego from what remains. Here we encounter a biological analogy:

> This is similar to the phenomena noted in the ingenious attempts of Jacques Loeb to stimulate unfertilized eggs to development by the action of chemicals, i.e. without fertilization: the chemicals disorganize the outer layers of the egg, but out of the detritus a protective bladder (sheath) is formed, which puts a stop to further injury. In the same way the Eros liberated by instinctual defusion converts destruction into growth, into a further development of the parts that have been protected.
>
> (Ferenczi, 1926a, p. 377)

As he notes four years later, in a short piece on 'Trauma and Striving for Health' (1930c), fragmentation as a result of trauma does not appear to be a sort of mechanical consequence of shock, but instead it is a form of defence, an adaptation. Here, he makes another analogy with lower animals who, subjected to extreme stimulation, break up and continue their existence in fragments. He goes on to imagine the logic of a defence by splitting (Ferenczi, 1930c). Fragmentation might prove useful to the subject because it creates a bigger surface open to the external world, increasing the possibility of discharging the many and unbearable affects of the scene of trauma. Fragmentation is also advantageous because it can dissolve the sense of unified perception. It is often the case that the suffering experienced in the scene of trauma is so great that the subject could not survive it. Splitting into pieces means that 'single fragments suffer for themselves; the unbearable unification of all pain qualities and quantities does not take place' (Ferenczi, 1930c, pp. 230–231). The integration of all pain would be the equivalent of psychic death.

By remaining on the productive borderline between creation and destruction – or by remaining curious about the fusion and defusion of the life drive and the death drive – Ferenczi authors a kind of 'psychoanalysis of organs' that takes seriously the organ (including newly formed organs) as a site of anxiety and signification and investigates the fascinating semi-autonomous qualities of organs to re-shape and re-fashion themselves into new formations. Some version of a psychoanalysis of organs takes shape in Ferenczi's writings of 1919, 1926, and 1932, where he introduces ideas such as 'organ neurosis' (1926b) and even more curious phenomena such as 'organ individuality' (1924, p. 82) or the 'cooperation of organs' (1924, p. 82). Organs appear to have a secret life: they are capable of different kinds of regressions, perversions, strangulations, condensations, displacements, doublings, which we usually attribute to the psychic stratum (Wilson, 2015).

We enter a clinical imagery of 'wise organs', or, as Ferenczi states: 'when the psychic system fails, the organism begins to think' (1932a, p. 6). The accent here is on the productive and materialising force of hysteria: the lump in the throat of the hysteric patient is not merely a hallucination, but it is part of a new 'grammar' of organs, a stirring up of the tissues of the throat, or of the contents of the stomach, or of the intestinal matter, which implies a capacity for condensation, displacement, repetition, or identification. This showcasing of the creativities of the hysterical symptom has important implications for how we can imagine the relationship between the psyche and the soma. In short, there is a 'horizontalising' gesture here, where the soma is just as capable of complex acts as the psyche.

In *Thalassa*, Ferenczi (1924, p. 82) talks about an internal qualitative differentiation in the sphere of the libido which can lead to an 'organ libido' and even an 'organ individuality'. As he writes:

> According to the 'theory of genitality', the cooperation of organs and of their component parts does not consist simply of the automatic adding together of useful workmen to give a sum total of performance. Each organ possesses a certain 'individuality'; in each and every organ there is repeated that conflict between ego- and libidinal interests which, too, we have encountered hitherto only in the analysis of *psychic individualities*.
>
> (Ferenczi, 1924, p. 83)

Ferenczi differentiates between the 'altruistic' functioning of organs and autoerotic or self-gratifying processes in the tissues. Organs are thus capable of cooperation, but this is not a guaranteed outcome; it takes struggle and a complicated negotiation between opposing forces. There is another image of radical plasticity of the psyche that is crucial here: Ferenczi describes a kind of layering of organs. It appears that, in the moment of trauma, '[n]ewly created organs in respect to their functions are only superposed upon the old without destroying them; even when the new functions make use of the material medium of the old, the latter organisation or function, although apparently given up, remains "potential", "biologically unconscious", and may again become active under certain circumstances' (Ferenczi, 1924, p. 93, fn). This layering or superimposition of organs means that any idea of evolution is questioned. The layered organs contain many temporalities within themselves, many references to other moments, including other catastrophes. It is a concentricity of catastrophes, where forward movement or progress will almost certainly involve a level of denial of this multiplicity of temporal references.

The connections that Ferenczi makes between destruction, creativity and the creation of new organs should not, however, seduce us into a celebration of fragments, a sort of enthusiasm for a post-catastrophic subjectivity. Ferenczi remains lucid on the dark implications of splitting, which pass through a particular kind of narcissism in which the deadened fragments of the ego are denied. The ego becomes a kind of mosaic of dead and still-alive parts, but the deadened and de-libidinised ones are 'forgotten'. Some of the fragments 'assume, as it were, the form and function of a whole person' (Ferenczi, 1930b, p. 222). Here, Ferenczi construes another analogy with the animal world. As he writes in 'Child Analysis in the Analysis of Adults':

> I have been told little tales like the one about the wicked animal which tries to destroy a jelly-fish by means of its teeth and claws, but cannot get at it because the jelly-fish with its subtleness eludes each jab and bite and then returns to its round shape. This story may be interpreted in two ways: on the one hand it expresses the passive resistance with which the patient meets the attacks of his environment, and on the other it represents the splitting of the self into a suffering, brutally destroyed part and a part which, as it were, knows everything but feels nothing.
>
> (Ferenczi, 1931a, p. 135)

The attention to the jellyfish brings a reminder of both the creative and destructive dimensions of catastrophe. The jellyfish, critter of the sea, is radically plastic during the attack. It re-becomes round, avoiding death. But at the same time, it momentarily dies, frozen in a passive state that mimics death. Paradoxically, the jellyfish survives because it has the ability to get closest to death.

In the analytic situation, the traces of this sort of splitting resurface when the patient feels hurt and disappointed, and as a result 'he starts playing by himself like a lonely child' (ibid). In some instances, parts of the body – hands, fingers, feet, genitals, head, nose, or eye – become 'representatives' of the entire person (ibid). The tragic pain of the scene of trauma is re-enacted using these body parts. This re-enactment, in the analytic situation, is equivalent to striving for a better solution to the one found at the time of the trauma. This gives us an insight into the precise and non-arbitrary nature of the symptom: very particular parts of the body are selected for the symptom, and they are tied to exact details of the trauma scene.

Ferenczi's biological analogies allow him to extend his trauma theory and to observe that new faculties emerge at the time of the trauma. This opens new paths in psychoanalytic theory in terms of how we think about repair and how the 'new organs' created in traumatic times can be part of this repair. In the 30 July 1932 entry of his *Clinical Diary*, Ferenczi (1932a, p. 181) concludes:

> A neoformation of the self is impossible without the previous destruction, either partial or total, or dissolution of the former self. A new ego cannot be formed directly from the previous ego, but from *fragments*, more or less elementary products of its disintegration. (Splitting, atomization.)

Neo-formations also bring neo-times, or new forms of temporal experience, sometimes disjunct and desynchronised from one another, sometimes deeply synchronised. The very idea of a cooperation of organs can be imagined in temporal terms as a synchronising of fragments into an ensemble. This synchronic experience is, however, fragile and precarious, and there is always a danger of falling into radically desynchronised times of organs, where each organ egoistically functions by itself and for itself, in its own time.

On Teleplastia

The 'new organs' produced at the time of the trauma emerge in a sudden manner. They are psychic events. It is a kind of 'teleplastic' transformation (Ferenczi, 1932a, p. 117), producing ad hoc organs that become responsible for some of the organism's functions. Teleplasty is another term that is key to Ferenczi's eventful psychoanalysis. In the *Clinical Diary*, he shows that in some cases the hallucination of breathing can maintain life, even where there is total somatic suffocation. It is as if the subject generates ex-corporated lungs, which are the teleplastic double of the physical lungs. For the purposes of defence and survival, the subject can also generate 'receptacles, gripping tools, tools of aggression' (Ferenczi, 1932a, p. 117) which will still fight for life, although the organism can find itself in a lifeless state or in deep coma.

To further concretise this intriguing idea of teleplasty, Ferenczi evokes the case of R.N., Elizabeth Severn, who imagined an infinitely expandable bladder formed at the back of her head where all her pain could accumulate (Ferenczi, 1932a, p 121). This pain-collecting bladder had a function in surviving the intensity of suffering in the scene of trauma. Ferenczi pays close attention in his clinical work to such odd organs, swelling up and disintegrating in relation to some detail of the scene. Among these odd organs, the protective bladder has a special place, allowing some partial and hallucinatory integration in a psychic time where the danger of complete disintegration looms.

Ferenczi discusses the task of the analyst in relation to such curious protective bladders. One of the tasks is to re-fashion the bladder from its fragments after it has burst or is shattered. Another task is to ensure that the bladder thus reconstructed is linked up with other parts of the ego and thus ceases to exist in complete isolation. The analyst is never above this scene of fragments and organs, having mastery over the scene, but somehow beside it, lateral to it. In terms of temporality, the analyst experiments with attuning herself to the times of these odd organs, bladders and fragments.

The Carp and the Tube

> *With each feeding, I got the growing feeling that it was my flesh the carp wanted. I began losing weight. After the fish had gobbled their lunch, I could not touch a bite of mine.*
>
> *At night, in my bed, the darkness around me was filled with gaping mouths. I put my head under the pillow in terror and cried. I could feel their obese, scaly, writhing bodies under the covers with me, suffocating me – their cold, smacking lips moving all over me.*
>
> *Jonah at least was lucky enough to be safely tucked away in the whale's stomach. Being swallowed by the carp wouldn't have been so bad. It wasn't their stomachs that terrified me, it was their mouths – the glottal vibrating of their mandibles sucking away at me, night after interminable night. My nightmare visions were not of fairies and castles but of creatures from Hieronymus Bosch.*
>
> *Related to this was the paralysing fear that if I endured too many of their loathsome kisses I would turn into one of them. I would become cylindrical. My hands explored my body, expecting to find tell-tale signs of this dreaded metamorphosis.*
>
> (Nothomb, 2000, p. 117)

In this short excerpt of Amélie Nothomb's novel *The Character of Rain*, what is fleshed out is a Ferenczian organ neurosis in which the protagonist's stomach becomes overinvested and gains autonomous functioning, de-synchronising itself from her other organs. While watching voracious carp feeding, she develops a fixation on the emptiness of her own stomach as a counterpoint to the anxiety-generating fullness of the fish. She suffers a metamorphosis and becomes-cylinder, retaining nothing from the outside and letting everything pass through. This curious transformation references a previous early moment in the character's life when, as a newborn baby, she experienced herself as a 'tube'. As Nothomb (2000, pp. 2–3) writes: 'There have been theories about tubes, and for a good reason: they are singular combinations of fullness and emptiness; they are hollow substance, a something that contains nothing. Tubes can be flexible, but it renders them no less mysterious'.

This scene of feeding the fish removes our character to another psychic time and to multiple scenes of being a vulnerable baby, being fed by her caregivers, while feeling unable to retain anything within herself. Everything passed through her – or through her-as-a-tube – in a way that was both devastating and liberating. Reviving the traumatic aspects of being fed, this new scene, where she is watching the food disappearing into the stomachs of the voracious fish, transforms her own stomach into a well-known shape of a cylinder. And she is now possessed by the image of being devoured by the carp and even by the prospect of becoming-carp. The 'stomach neurosis' constitutes a regression to the earlier state that Nothomb (2000, pp. 2–3) calls 'cylindrical serenity – filtering everything in the universe, retaining nothing'.

In the consulting room, the analytical orientation towards this stomach neurosis would be to listen to the organ's 'voice' and its time, attempting some form of synchronisation with the time of the organ. The analyst would strive to learn the language of the organ, which includes references to and images of gaping mouths, smacking lips, vibrating mandibles and tubular and cylindrical shapes.

Orpha and the Eternal Present

Analysands play a very important part in creating psychoanalytic knowledge, and this often remains unacknowledged and bears no inscription. In his book *Elizabeth Severn: The 'Evil Genius' of Psychoanalysis*, psychoanalyst Arnold W. Rachman traces the encounter between Ferenczi and one of his key patients, Elizabeth Severn, who is also the protagonist of the *Clinical Diary*. In Rachman's account, Ferenczi and his patient Severn appear as a creative dyad. What we usually regard as Ferenczi's 'trauma theory' is treated as a co-creation. Without Severn's experimentations with self-hypnotic trance states, Ferenczi would perhaps not have fully grasped the importance of regression and reliving in the psychoanalytic frame or the importance of the analysis of countertransference.

There is another question that opens here. Our writing, as psychoanalytic authors, is *full* of our patients, and we are yet to invent forms of thinking and writing to traverse this particular kind of fullness. We could speak of a *co-montage of the psychoanalytic dyad*, where various heterogeneous elements hold together in a new constellation, or composition, or ensemble. The psychoanalytic process is a co-production, a co-affectation, a coalition. A part of its elements come from the patient, a part from the analyst, and a part are co-created in the encounter between the two. The elements can be dreams, free-associations, fantasies, metaphors and symbolisations. This singular constellation determines what kind of psychoanalytic theory gets written, usually by the psychoanalyst in the dyad, who thus operates as the one that transcribes what is fundamentally a co-creation.

The relationship between Ferenczi and Elizabeth Severn has been looked at by psychoanalysts and historians such as Christopher Fortune (1993), Martin Stanton (1991), Benjamin Wolstein (1992), Arnold W. Rachman (2017), Nancy A. Smith (1998), and Peter Rudnytsky (2017, 2021). Notably, Christopher Fortune (1993) conducted an important investigation to establish the identities of the cases present in the *Clinical Diary*, which are marked there by initials. Elizabeth Severn appears in the *Diary* with the initials R.N.

Elizabeth Severn was born as Leota Loretta Haywood in Milwaukee, Wisconsin, in the United States, in 1879. Between the ages of 18 months and 11 years, she was the subject of repeated sexual abuse perpetrated by her father. This led to psychic splitting and severe states of dissociation. This complex traumatic state led Severn to be admitted to a psychiatric institution for a period of two years, following a 'breakdown' that occurred a year after her marriage ended in 1905. During her short marriage, Severn gave birth to a daughter, Margaret, who later became an internationally renowned dancer and with whom Severn maintained a close relationship throughout her lifetime (Rachman, 2017). Following her discharge from the psychiatric institution, Severn continued to suffer from a range of symptoms that included confusion, hallucinations, nightmares and suicidal depression. Given these enduring symptoms, she searched for a variety of remedies and forms of release, which included seeing a theosophically minded physician. This therapeutic encounter is connected to Severn's inclination to pursue the path of a 'healer'. This is how she started her own experimentations with therapeutic roles and even advertised herself as a 'metaphysician' and 'psychotherapist', as Rachman (2017) documents. Apart from seeing patients, Severn also experimented with her voice as an author and published several of her writings. Perhaps the most notable is *The Discovery of the Self: A Study of Psychological Cure* (1933), republished in 2017 with an important introductory note by Peter Rudnytsky in which he contextualises the book and offers further insights into the complex relationship between Severn and Ferenczi.

By 1924, Severn had made several attempts to start a psychoanalytic process with American analysts, but all of these explorations failed as she continued to experience dissociative states, migraines, exhaustion and suicidal depression. Importantly, she had little or no recollection of her life prior to the age of twelve. Following advice from Otto Rank, she relocated from the United States to Budapest so as to start her analysis with Ferenczi. Notably, Ferenczi was well-known in psychoanalytic circles of the time as the analyst of very difficult patients (Bonomi, 2015/II, p. 201) and as a therapist who accepted cases that other analysts had not seen good results with. They were often patients in states that we would nowadays refer to as traversing borderline states (Green, 1996) or even patients traversing psychotic states. While in Budapest, Severn embarked on an eight-year analytic process with Ferenczi, which continued until close to Ferenczi's death when he could no longer work.

*

Let us get closer to Elizabeth Severn, and to the complex transferential relationship between Severn and Ferenczi, through one of her dreams about psychic fragmentation that Ferenczi analyses in his *Clinical Diary*. Severn's dreams are often very striking, nearly nightmarish sequences of images, where aggression, violation, breakdown of communication and the impossibility of linking disparate parts are recurrent themes. But these dreams are also 'helpers' to the analysis, allowing the analyst to have a sense of the character of the different fragments, their respective forms of defence and their relationships to one another.

One of the most important Ferenczian revisions to Freud's ideas on dreams is the great weight given to the traumatolytic function of the dream. This means that the dream is the place of return for unmastered traumatic sensory impressions which struggle for a (better) solution. The dreams that Ferenczi writes about are thus accounts of complicated scenes of psychic fragmentation. They are also tied up with the reparative repetition that I discussed in a previous section of the book: through dreams, the impressions inscribed in the register of memory of the id can gain form.

Let us step into the dream:

> R.N.: frequently recurring form of dream: two, three, or even several persons represent, according to the completed dream-analysis, an equal number of component parts of her personality. The dream analysed today, for instance, was dramatized as follows: the dreamer herself receives a written message from the beloved person who is closest to her, which reads: 'Here I am. I am here.' The dreamer attempts to tell this to a third person, a man, but she can contact him only indirectly, by a long-distance telephone call, and in fact the whole conversation with this man sounds very indistinct, as if coming from an immense distance. The difficulty increases to the point of a nightmarish and helpless struggle because of the fact that the text of the message cannot be read directly; the dreamer sees it only in mirror-writing, as light shines through the postcard; she is sitting in a kind of tent, and can see the writing only as mirror-writing.
>
> (Ferenczi, 1932a, p. 157)

One of the key images here is that of an agonising breakdown of communication. As Ferenczi (1932a, p. 158) writes in his interpretation of the dream, 'this personality, shattered and made defenseless by suffering and poison, is attempting, over and over again but always unsuccessfully, to reassemble its various parts into a unit, that is, to understand the event taking place in and around her'. Integration is impossible and the psychic life of fragments is marked by confusion and distortion. The dream even records the impossibility of direct representation by reference to 'mirror writing', a painful and inversed inscription in need of a transposition before the message can be understood. The radical splitting of various parts of the psyche is symbolised as the long-distance telephone call and an 'immense distance'. The

'I' of the dream, perhaps standing for the conscious ego, is unable to deliver the written messages. The fragments are linked to one another in a precarious way (if at all), and the connection can collapse at any point.

In his interpretation of this dream, Ferenczi does not, however, explore its transferential dimensions. What could this dream tell us about the transference between Severn and Ferenczi? Could it be that Severn experienced some aspects of the analysis itself as a form of 'mirror writing', some difficult inscription that is laboursome and that can also break down easily? While this is a speculative idea, it links up with something that transpires in the *Clinical Diary* itself and in Severn's correspondence (Rachman, 2017): her analysis knew many impasses and challenges. Ferenczi and Severn also notoriously experimented with mutual analysis, which means that at a certain point in Severn's analysis, when the process seemed very stuck, after insistence from Severn, the two agreed to 'swap' roles, which meant that they would take turns being in the role of analyst and patient. This unusual development was also possible because Ferenczi came to think that his own analysis (with Freud) was unfinished and that this fact influenced his analytic position with Severn. There were significant unanalysed 'remainders' from his analysis with Freud that meant some of his early traumatic experiences remained unsymbolised and unelaborated. Freud was in principle weary of regressive states and, through his own analytical posture of cold neutrality, did not enable Ferenczi to get in touch with these more regressed remnants of his own scene of trauma. These 'remnants' forcefully came to the fore in the analysis with Elizabeth Severn, which was very demanding for Ferenczi. He slowly came to realise that he had an inhibition and even aversion in relation to strong female figures, which remitted him to the position of being a young, vulnerable and perhaps overstimulated boy who received confusing seductive messages from a governess who was caring for him at the time.

Let us recall how Ferenczi writes in the *Diary* about his residue from the analysis with Freud:

> My own analysis could not be pursued deeply enough because of my analyst (by his own admission, of a narcissistic nature), with his strong determination to be healthy, and his antipathy toward any weaknesses, or abnormalities, could not follow me down into those depths, and introduced the 'educational' stage too soon. Just as Freud's strength

> lies in the firmness of education, mine lies in the depth of the relaxation technique.
>
> (Ferenczi, 1932a, p. 62)

This acknowledgement of the impasses in the analysis Ferenczi had with Freud is relevant because it stimulates Ferenczi to develop his ideas on the importance of the analyst's working on their own countertransference: the analyst needs to be committed to constantly addressing the more regressive aspects of the psyche which are bound to be stirred up by certain engagements with patients and which need to be kept in check and elaborated in the analyst's own analysis, in their supervision, their self-analysis and clinical reflections. It is from this observation that Ferenczi could ramify his own vocabulary on analytical tact and sensitivity, on the professional hypocrisy of the analyst, on the potential retraumatising valency of the psychoanalytic process, if the analyst will repeat the forms of denial that the patient suffered as a child.

Ferenczi went into the 'mutual analysis' experiment with Elizabeth Severn in a hesitant, even reluctant manner. This reluctance and the dilemmatic states that led to the decision to give in to the patient's demand of alternating the roles of patient and analyst are recorded in the *Clinical Diary*. To the reader, it seems that this clinical experiment took place out of some tragic necessity rather than out of any desire to enrich clinical technique, or to push boundaries, or to stimulate theoretical and clinical innovations. It is interesting to follow the trace of Ferenczi's reservations and struggles with mutual analysis and its implications which are recorded in entries of the *Diary*, such as: 'Mutual analysis and the *limits* of its application' (entry of 17 January 1932); 'A *dilemma* of mutual analysis' (entry of 2 February 1932); '*Limitations* of mutual analysis' (entry of 16 February 1932); '*Transformation* of mutual analysis into simply being analysed' (entry of 29 March 1932); 'Unconscious *struggle* of sensitivities between patient and analyst' (entry of 3 May 1932); and 'Advantages and disadvantages, that is, optimal *limits* of countertransference' (entry of 6 July 1932) – emphases mine. Indeed, having been through the depths of the mutual analysis experience, Ferenczi (1932a, p. 115) concludes: 'Mutual analysis: only a last resort! Proper analysis by a stranger, without any obligation, would be better'.

In the *Diary*, we are offered a moment of self-analysis when Ferenczi articulates some important threads of his own scene of trauma. The remainders of the scene of trauma were revivified in the transference to Elizabeth Severn. A series of psychic images came into focus for him, all having to do with the disproportionate and seductive powers of a female figure in relation to him as a boy-child. This is how Ferenczi accounts for his antipathy and even recoiling in relation to (strong) female figures, which functioned as a defence in relation to his early seduction:

> the patient felt the irritation and the resistance, and this is what had led her to propose mutual analysis. […] I submerged myself deeply into the reproduction of infantile experiences; the most evocative image was the vague appearance of female figure, probably servant girls from earliest childhood; then the image of a corpse, whose abdomen I was opening up, presumably in the dissecting room; linked to this the mad fantasy that I was pressed into this wound in the corpse. Interpretation: the after-effect of passionate scenes, which presumably did take place, in the course of which the housemaid probably allowed me to play with her breasts, but then pressed my head between her legs, so that I became frightened and felt I was suffocating. This is the source of my hatred of females: I was to dissect them for it, that is to kill them. This is why my mother's accusation: 'You are my murderer' cut to the heart and led to (1) a compulsive desire to help anyone who is suffering, especially women; and (2) a flight from situations in which I would have been aggressive.
>
> (Ferenczi, 1932a, pp. 60–61)

Ferenczi was thus traumatically inclined to show a 'superkindness' (1932a, p. 86) in relation to Severn while actually feeling an unelaborated dislike for her. This form of unconscious 'hypocrisy' functioned as a form of denial and was a potential source of re-traumatisation for Severn, who – being herself endowed with a traumatically enhanced emphatic capacity – could sense that there were some conflicted, untrue, or negated aspects in the countertransference. Ultimately, Ferenczi's 'superkindness' or 'superperformance' was a manifestation of analytic guilt for not being able to like her or help her sufficiently with her suffering. This created a blockage in the psychoanalytic process which we can arguably attribute – not without risking oversimplification of an intricate relationship – to Ferenczi's particular 'troubles' in the countertransference to Severn.

Despite these troubles in transference and countertransference, I believe the Ferenczi-Severn dyad left an important legacy. In the opening entry of the *Diary*, Ferenczi acknowledges the ramifications of the powerful mutual analysis experiment and reports that 'the communication of the content of my own psyche developed into a form of mutual analysis, from which I, the analyst, derived much profit' (Ferenczi, 1932a, p. 3), while in his closing entry he records Severn's hope that what will remain of their joint work 'is a reciprocal "honorable" recognition of mutual achievement' (Ferenczi, 1932a, p. 214).

Today we are in the position to reconstitute, through the *Clinical Diary* and also through archival material related to Elizabeth Severn's life and work, that she played a very active part in making sense of her own state of psychic fragmentation. In particular, she is the one who coined the term 'Orpha' to name the psychic position of watching herself from above or from afar while parts of the psyche are in agony, as if the suffering parts were an 'other'. Ferenczi took further steps in understanding such phenomena of self-care and, on the basis of his rich experience with difficult cases, he concluded that Orphic phenomena are ubiquitous: we are all susceptible to Orphic functioning, although to a larger or smaller degree depending on our singular state of psychic fragmentation. What we all share is the capacity to generate a fragment that cares for the other parts of the psyche when the expectations of any external help have failed and when suffering becomes unbearable. It is significant to name the fact that Severn named Orpha so as to counter the trend of what Arnold W. Rachman (2017, p. 57) refers to as *Todschweigen* or 'death by silence', understood as the disowning of a psychoanalytic dissident by suppressing and censoring them in order to preserve mainstream psychoanalytic thought and practice. There are sufficient traces to consider that Severn was an analyst in training, an author and creator in her own right, and the co-author of some of Ferenczi's insights on trauma and regression, and not just a 'difficult case' that Ferenczi treated.

This short contextualisation of the experiment of mutual analysis of the Ferenczi-Severn dyad opens a question that has ramifications for the contemporary clinic: how to understand *mutuality* in the psychoanalytic process? And what are the technical implications of becoming starkly aware of the *hierarchical* nature of the psychoanalytic process, where the analyst is in a position of strength while the patient can be fixed in a position of powerlessness, vulnerability, and even infantilised? How can the psychoanalytic relationship be *horizontalised*, with effective clinical interventions and beyond the illusion of a perfectly democratised relationship between two equals? Ferenczi was profoundly aware that, for any fleeting moment of horizontality in the psychoanalytic frame to take place, an intervention of horizontalising the relationship needs to occur – and that it can occur only if it can be sustained by the analyst. It is not a rare occurrence that due to narcissistic conflict the analyst is unable to initiate or sustain this horizontality. They cannot see themselves as a subject of trauma and regression, similar to the patient. In this context, the analysis of the analyst becomes crucial, and it was Ferenczi who was the first to state this in very clear and uncompromising terms. As he writes: 'The best analyst is the patient who has been cured' and 'Analysts should be analysed *better*, *not* worse, than patients' (Ferenczi, 1932a, p. 115). If this is not the case, and the analyst has significant narcissistic residues from their own analysis, they are at risk of occupying a position of denial in the analysis and even of being cruel and sadistic to the patient, and thus retraumatising them.

The analysis of the analyst and the constant analysis of the countertransference are crucial because they are oriented towards eliminating obstacles to the treatment that originate in the analyst's psychic functioning. The position of the analyst must thus first and foremost be *different* from the situation of childhood, or from the scene of trauma, which would have been one of suggestion and of the emergence of infantile obedience and submission. In the *Clinical Diary*, Ferenczi (1932a, p. 38) writes that mutuality is 'an antidote against the hypnotic lies in childhood'. By taking a different position, and by practising recognition where denial used to be, the analyst can become a vehicle of 'demechanisation' or 'dehypnotising' (Ferenczi, 1932a, p. 63). This means that the analysand gradually reinstates the trust in their own senses and no longer feels the need to submit to an overpowering force that tells them what to do and what to think. Their relation to power and authority can be substantially reconfigured.

*

The psychic processes described so far – from 'getting beside oneself' and the ex-corporation of the ego, to 'traumatic progression' and the sudden maturation of a part of the psyche – all constitute what I would call Orphic functioning or Orphic phenomena. As I pointed out, these splitting processes are forms of *narcissistic splitting*. Under the strength of the traumatic attack, the psyche is forced to devise new ways to care for itself, and at times the only way to do so is by fragmenting itself and producing a 'scene' of care internally, populated by distinct parts of the psyche that act like 'carers' and other parts that act like those to be 'cared for'. The self treats one of its parts as an 'other' and takes *it* as an object.

Orpha is one of the most fascinating results of this narcissistic splitting. It is more than a mere mechanism of defence: I argue that we can treat Orpha as a new psychic agency, a fourth agency alongside the id, ego and superego. In the *Clinical Diary*, we come across an entire vocabulary that allows us to imagine the psychic life of Orpha. Some remarkable terms of this new Orphic vocabulary are: 'guardian angel' (1932a, pp. 8–10 & pp. 102–106); 'ancient substitute (to thinking)'; 'substitute mother' (1932a, pp. 102–106); 'dissociation of fragments and organs'; 'explosion'; 'destruction of psychic associations'; 'anarchy of organs (where reciprocal cooperation is compromised)' (1932a, pp. 68–70).

Orpha is the result of traumatic self-caring, defending the psyche from sensations of unbearable intensity of the scene of trauma. Orpha is the form that the organising life instincts take at the time of the trauma, precisely when the enormity of suffering has resulted in a renunciation of any expectation of external help. As Ferenczi (1932a, p. 105) notes, '[t]he absent external help [...] is replaced by the creation of a more ancient substitute'. Orpha is a sort of 'guardian angel', a healing agent, and a principle of salvation: by surprising, minute calculations about what it would mean to continue living (often in a basic sense of continuing breathing or maintaining a beating heart), Orpha acts in the direction of self-preservation. We often encounter such minute calculations in instances when a person preserves their life, despite all odds, in circumstances of extreme strain. Imagine an air-tight small room, where someone is locked up by their aggressor. How little air can they breathe in, in order to postpone reaching the end of their air supply and increase the chances of being found by carers returning home from work? Orphic functioning means that a part of the self produces an improbable answer to such an apparently irresolvable puzzle and regulates the breathing, ensuring that the air supply lasts exactly until the anticipated time of return of the saviours. Furthermore, in the clinical realm, in the countertransference, the presence of Orpha often creates for the analyst a reaction of surprise at the very event of survival in such improbable circumstances. It is as if a question forms: 'How did my patient survive this terrible attack!?'

Orpha also 'produces wish-fulfilling hallucinations, consolation phantasies; it anaesthetises the consciousness and sensitivity against sensations as they become unbearable' (Ferenczi, 1932a, p. 8). What is remarkable here is that with Orpha any dichotomy between reason and passion collapses. Orpha is created by the intrusion of the language of passion in the realm of the language of tenderness. Orpha is wise but it is a fragment, split-off from other faculties. It is formed when death is very near, yet it acts as an organising life instinct.

As I see it, Orpha brings an account of the emergence of hyper-faculties and of over-performance. A strange product of the traumatic shock, Ferenczi writes, Orpha manifests itself as 'an unperturbed intelligence which is not restricted by any chronological or spatial resistances in its relation to the environment' (Ferenczi, 1931b, pp. 245–246). As I noted, the construction of Orpha is based to a large extent on the analysis of Elizabeth Severn/patient R.N. Ferenczi records a series of trans-human images that R.N. shares with him in the analysis. She experiences sensations of exploding into the universe, accompanied by images of shining constellations. She is populated by hallucinatory phrases, such as 'I am the universal egg'. This enigmatic image points to a fantasy that she is the centre of the world and has incorporated the entire universe within herself (Ferenczi, 1932a, p. 29). Ordinary 'human' space and time referents here lose their meaning.

Orpha is also a metapsychologically plausible account of a particular kind of clairvoyance. On the couch, Orpha appears as a fragment of the psyche that sometimes instructs, directs or guides the analyst with great precision as to what to do, how to speak, how to be silent, in order to allow the reliving of the traumatic sequence of events. As Ferenczi writes in the *Clinical Diary*, commenting on the analysis of R.N., 'At her demand and insistence, I help her by asking simple questions that compel her to think. I must address her as if she were a patient in a mental hospital, using her childhood nicknames, and force her to admit to the reality of the facts, in spite of their painful nature' (1932a, p. 14). We would be tempted to believe in the first instance that such instructions or demands coming from the patient are a form of resistance; in moments of reliving the scene of trauma, and for structuring of Orphic functioning, such forms of 'guidance' are a resonance of Orphic hyper-faculties. In a sense, Orpha knows what can't be known by way of regular faculties of reason and logical understanding.

An Orphic time is one when individuals become aware of their hyper-faculties and are able to use them for the benefit of others, not only for narrow self-interest. 'For the visionary adult', Ferenczi writes (1931b, pp. 244–245), 'the infantile amnesia disappears, and, due to the lifting of the barriers of repression, he is able to establish communication with the visionary child, and the capacities of the latter stay with the adult'.

The many children populating Ferenczi's work, with Orpha as a central figure, align themselves as the messengers of a kind of sensorial messianism. After the scene of trauma, some of the psychic fragments resulting from traumatic splitting gain semi-autonomous lives; they become curious 'sites' for hyper-faculties. Like Orpheus's head after his death, they are both dead – since they have become separated from the body – and alive – since they can function as an oracle and open a window onto the future. Part of the Orphic omnipotence is an acute sense of anticipation. Orpha contains all possible futures in the present when she decides over her own fate and the fate of the others. When expectations are not met, a new form of denial ensues. Orpha has already decided on how things will unfold, and any amendment to this decision is unimaginable.

Let us recall Ovid's myth of Orpheus. Orpheus is the son of Muse Calliope, 'of the beautiful voice', and of a mortal father, Oiagros, a Thracian king 'who hunts all alone' (Kerényi, 1959, p. 280). Orpheus is a poet who, with his gift of the lyre, descends on his own into the Underworld, into 'Persephone's sad realm', to bind Eurydice in love. As Kerényi tells us, Orpheus's name is related to *orphne* – a sombre garment that Orpheus wore when he made sacrifice to Hecate on behalf of the Argonauts; it thus stands for darkness and gloom. Indeed, Orpheus lives between the luminous beauty of the lyre and this sombre garment. We also know that Apollo was Orpheus's divine father and that he offered him his lyre, while it was the Muses who taught him how to play it (Graves, 1992). The music of Orpheus's lyre was unlike that of any mortal: when he played, trees would be drawn to him, wild animals were tamed, and the inhabitants of the Underworld became uncharacteristically moved by feelings of compassion for others. Orpheus went along with the Argonauts on their journey to obtain the Golden Fleece and the magical sound of his lyre drowned the Sirens' song. After Eurydice's untimely death, he descends into the

Underworld to save her, but because he fails to keep to the condition of not looking back at her during the journey, Eurydice returns to the dead, while Orpheus's lyre fails him, and he is unable to enter the Underworld again to bring her back. When Orpheus dies, his body becomes dismembered, but, as ancient writers tell us, his head is enshrined and survives as an oracle, separated from the body.

Within the myth of Orpheus, our focus is precisely on the death of Orpheus and on his dismemberment. Orpheus's head is a tragic fragment, both dead and alive. It is alive in the sense of being able to contribute in a striking, improbable, clairvoyant way to the collective life, by way of a hyper-faculty.

What emerges from here is a novel, non-Oedipal clinical and theoretical imaginary. A kind of Orphic register. Nancy Smith (1999, p. 345) marks the difference between the Oedipal register and the Orphic register: '[the myth of Oedipus] throbs with conflict, murderous aggression, incest, and guilt', while '[t]he Orpheus and Eurydice myth, in contrast to the Oedipus myth, aches with fragmentation, separation, suffering due to acts of violation, as well as an attempt at reclamation motivated by love'. In this Orphic atmosphere, improbable survival meets deadly omnipotence.

I am very interested in the temporalities of the psychic fragment Orpha. I believe that Orpha produces a temporal effect in the psyche akin to that of living in an eternal present. It is an omnipotent, triumphant, flat temporality, where events cannot be enchained in a meaningful sequence, or tied into a line of imagined heritage or consequence, but they are experienced as stand-alone and severed from one another. Orpha's eternalised time is the time of gods, saviours and miracles, reminiscent of the time of survival in the scene of trauma, against all odds, when continuing living would have been an improbable event. Later in life, Orphic time preserves its omnipotence; it violently pulls the subject away from the reality principle and invites dangerous forms of overexertion – as if saying, 'I can do anything'.

Vignette: On Orphic Omnipotence

Val is a 34-year-old woman who came to analysis after a car accident, in which, all of a sudden, she felt pulverised into a cloud of particles, or, in her words, entirely 'up in the air'. In the first sessions, she also shared with me her incapacity to 'find her body' or to be in contact with it, in its material concreteness or fullness. She revealed to me that for years she exercised 'sustaining' her gaze and bearing being seen and gazed upon. Now she would manage to look people in the eye, including me, but to me it felt both too forward and too withdrawn, somewhat artificial and rehearsed, betraying her attempts at mastering the gaze, rather than her actually being able to access a form of intimate contact between people.

Val is extremely bright and has many talents (from musical composition to playing musical instruments to writing poetry). She is a very intense presence in the session. In the first year of her analysis, I often found myself tensing my own muscles, or holding my hands together tightly, as if there was a need to secure a tremendous force. Val works partly as a sports instructor. This revealed itself to be her own route into finding out what it is to have a body or even her own research into basic questions about bodies and body rhythms: how to breathe? how to feel your different muscles? and most of all, perhaps, how to relax your muscles?

There is a quality of her 'thinking through' things (her own actions, her relationship to others) that feels like a material taking-things-apart, or undoing things. It feels more like dissecting than thinking. It is sharp and always has an 'edge', but it is also detached from its object. It is indeed a hyper-thinking, which reminds me of Ferenczi's comparison between the faculties of the wise baby and the premature ripening of a fruit that was bitten by a bird.

Val lost her mother early on in her life, when she was still a baby. She was cared for by a distant relative, an aunt, called Nina. There are reasons to believe that Val's caregiving aunt had a psychotic structure. A descendant of immigrants, she refused to learn the language of her host country at the time (an Asian country), and she always spoke English to Val, creating somewhat of a private linguistic bubble around them. She also insisted on home-schooling Val. Nina would often have episodes of 'agony', when she would lock herself in her room and come out only after several days with a completely unpredictable mood. Val felt abandoned and was often in the position to care of herself, while also making superhuman efforts to attune herself to the moods of her aunt.

A great deal of space is given in the analysis to understanding her being in an 'eternal present', where the intensity of the immediate 'now' trumps any possibility of imagining the future or planning the future, and any need to maintain an anchor into the past. It is an imperative, cruel present, as well as one that is glamorous and triumphant. In this elongated, unstoppable present, there is a very particular kind of 'testing' going on (I would say a kind of modified, post-traumatic 'reality testing'). Val will test herself all the time, giving herself the most astounding tasks, just to prove to herself she is capable of completing them. For a long time, she used to get involved in new sports activities that she had very little interest in, just so that she could test herself in new ways and stretch her abilities. She would also embark on radically new projects all the time, and although these would indeed look very interesting and creative in the 'eternal present', in her own life course they had the nature of 'undoing' her other achievements, damaging any possibility of giving some continuity to older projects, attacking any sense of an accumulation, or cumulative action, in which one act is leaning on another act, which in its turn is leaning on another act.

The very sentence: 'Let's see if I can do this' has a nearly hallucinatory power over her. She does not perform; she over-performs. I experience her faculties as hyper-faculties. This odd testing of limits has little to do, I believe, with superego imperatives or demands. Her 'tests' are not aimed at achieving social prestige, at being recognised, at abiding with some higher social or moral law, at emulating some role model, or at surpassing the achievements of her ancestors. The tests are rather a kind of repetition of a scene of survival in improbable or overwhelming circumstances. This is what the voice of the Ferenczian Orpha sounds like: it will utter, 'Let's see if I can do this' to the ego, taking the subject out of historical time and into an elongated, suspended, cruel present. We could say it will seduce the ego into over-exercising itself. There is no possibility of historical depth here or even of the temporality of the *Nachträglichkeit*; there is just a single flat surface which contains all the acts. Let us remember that Ferenczi describes Orpha as 'an unperturbed intelligence which is not restricted by any chronological or spatial resistances in its relation to the environment' (Ferenczi, 1931b, pp. 245–246).

But there is yet another facet to the very particular 'testing' that I am describing. Val will often 'test' others in the same way that she tests herself. As the tests are demanding and they take people out of their comfort zones and out of what is to be anticipated in the space of a given relationship, many people fail the tests, and they are thus 'dropped' in reality (as friends or meaningful connections) or degraded in fantasy as having revealed their unworthy nature. Val mentioned many instances where she derived enjoyment from throwing someone out of balance. After the first year of analysis, at a time when her analysis was going well as far as I could tell, she also 'tested' me in a similar way, coming into a session that was not far from the winter break and announcing that she had reflected on it, and she thought she would 'call off' the analysis after the break. In this instance, I passed the test, as my interpretation at the time was to state how sad I felt that she attached so little value to being in balance. It was a moment of great intensity and she did manage to cause me (and transmit to me) a sense of being thrown out of a state of balance, of being taken by surprise, while my reactions were being coldly observed and judged.

The Orpha fragment of the psyche is triumphant, since at the time of the trauma it triumphed over a near-deadly attack. Later in life, this psychic fragment insists on overcoming impossible obstacles it often manufactures for itself. Indeed, the near-deadly nature of the 'test' becomes a condition for libidinal satisfaction.

Val's Orphic states came from a place just as terrible as these actions announced. After the first year of treatment, Val told me about the existence of a 'secret', something that does not fit into words, something that she has been carrying around with her and she could not utter to anyone. In the countertransference, I felt something tremendous was being communicated. I acknowledged having received something of great importance, but I never asked a direct question about this terrible event.

After another year, Val told me her secret that stood beyond words. At around three years of age, while her aunt Nina was living an isolated and friendless life, Nina made Val a confidante and told her several of her life events. One event stood apart; it was like no other. When Nina was in her twenties, she was kidnapped by an older man, who assaulted her, left cigarette burn marks on her skin, and abandoned her in a distant location. The child was given a lot of details, including the atrocious scene of her aunt being burnt with the cigarette.

Val's Orpha is a result of having survived, abandoned by all external help, bearing witness to this particular story of sexual violence. The caregiver deposited in her something that she herself could not share with the adults around her, a great crushing 'secret' ridden with violence and abuse. The child was transfixed by the story of violence, both repellent and capable of producing arresting excitation. The 'enigma' of adult sexuality was presented to her alongside images of protruding into another person's body, breaking it apart, and burning it.

Val was bound to her caregiver, bearing her terrible secret. She was thus tied to an unspeakable scene of violence, where she is never in the position of the victim, for that place is already occupied by the aunt. She was also bound to the scene of violence through the many identifications that took place while incorporating this scene. She was identified with the humiliated and abused aunt. She was also identified with the attacker, always suspecting people (including herself) of being capable of committing acts of arbitrary violence. With this transmission, Nina and Val had a silent 'pact' of unidirectional and unconditional compassion. Nina was cast in the role of the victim of the violent past, so she was to be protected, spared from further aggression. While Nina continued over the years to make narcissistic use of Val, invading her and making implausible demands from her, Val's Orpha assembled as a phantasmatic triumph (and thus, a form of denial as well) over this very state of submission to the caregiver's wishes.

At the height of Orphic functioning, I would say that the 'gaze' is internal. A fragment is watching over the ego from the position of a guardian angel. With this, an internal effect of care is generated (I care for myself as if I were an other, in the absence of the care from an other), but at the cost of being able to hold another in my gaze or to gaze upon an other or to take an other as an object.

Narcissistic omnipotence of Orphic origin compromises one's ability to tell relative sizes. Orpha is unable to differentiate between big and small, important and unimportant, regular or catastrophic. The analyst's intervention takes on a kind of size-specifying function, allowing more and more differentiation and gradation of dimensions to take place. Orpha does not know of the size of the caregiver in relation to the child. Orpha does not know that 'your mother was big and you were small' or that 'you were smaller than your caregiver'. The punitive aspect of the superego (which is very loud and present in Orphic functioning) can make use of Orpha's lack of capacity to tell size, punishing the ego for not being able, as a three-year-old child, to 'save' the caregiver or to spare her of all her suffering. The interaction between the superego and Orpha is crucial to observe, here, and takes up a lot of the work of analysis. At times, patients in Orphic states tell me that I don't criticise them enough, or that I could be harsher with them, or push their limits more. This is a very important instance of the Orpha fragment of the psyche functioning in tandem with a punitive superego to achieve a unique form of 'internal sadism', where different aspects of the self are devising an arrangement in which they can torment each other and make the 'life' of the ego untenable.

In sum, interpretations where the 'fact of smallness' is repeated to the patient can lead to very positive results. When the traumatic scene is being described, the utterance by the analyst that 'you were small and therefore could not do more' often comes to the patient as a positive shock of relative sizes, a kind of revelation, as if the hallucinatory and omnipotent iterations, in which they are always great and powerful (or they should have been so), can stop. Interpretations about the size of things thus produce a surprising effect, and they stop the spiralling confusions between victims and perpetrators.

An important complication here occurs in cases, such as Val's, where the position of the victim is occupied by the aggressor in a very 'clever' way, involving a montage that is nearly perfectly concealed. The aunt managed to intrude into Val's psychic life precisely by presenting a message that she was the absolute victim, thus silently inverting the roles between the one who cares and the one who is being cared for.

I sometimes make interpretations that explicitly point to the state of the ego's being in fragments, such as: 'one part of you is making A, B and C demands from me, but I cannot side with it in this instance for X, Y and Z reasons'. In my experience, this produces a combination of tension and relaxation that is very productive for analytic work. Instead of fantasising about an unachievable wholeness, patients learn to think of themselves as a choir of voices, where some voices are at times working against the other ones. They thus learn a kind of internal suspicion, being weary of completely giving into the demands of a cruel, sadistic, omnipotent part of themselves.

Another important technical tool is an insistence on analogies. I am speaking here about the interpretation starting with 'this is just like when…'. Referencing particular episodes that the patient recounted to us, and making a parallel (often imperfect) to the episode currently narrated, is also crucial and produces a 'shock' on the even temporal surface of Orphic functioning, a 'shock' out of the eternal present and into a temporality that has more than one moment. The patient is gradually induced into a time with many 'knots', some of which have similarities. Ultimately, they perceive that these similarities are there because they have an ego which, although in fragments, does produce similar effects in the world, in different moments in time. Yet another analogy to draw is with childhood scenes. The analyst's interpretation that 'this makes me think of a child doing A, B and C' can initially outrage or wound an omnipotent Orphic voice, insisting on her eternal adulthood and on her being all-knowing, but gradually the patient learns to think of herself as 'also small' or 'sometimes small' and even to imagine that they were once a helpless child, and the burden of care and responsibility should have been, by all measure of reason, with their actual caregivers.

On Orphic Hyper-faculties

> *When he saw that Diane was seeking grand-motherly asylum, he told his elder sister that he would stay at home 'to stop Maman from eating Célia [the youngest sister] as if she were some coconut cake.'*
> *This was no mere image: Marie's excessive love for Célia evoked the swooning of certain thirteenth-century saints when swallowing the communion host. It was holy gluttony.*
>
> (Nothomb, 2017, p. 50)

The Orphic scene described here involved three siblings. The older sister, Diane, is fleeing to her grandmother's house to save herself from constant abandonment by the mother and its psychically deadening effect. To an extent, we have here an improbable act, one of revolt against lack of love, or against being dropped or abandoned, which is a rather unlikely psychic position. We might ask: where does the capacity for such a defiant psychic posture come from? Many 'dropped' children actually feel paralysed by the lack of love and less able than our character Diane to change their circumstances. But let us go further into the scene as it is described.

The younger brother remains behind with the mother and her newborn baby girl, Célia, because he is able to register the fact that the mother is devouring the baby girl with her love. The mother's love, very likely because of her own narcissistic wounds, is not calibrated to her children's need for love and care. For Diane, she had no love and attention: she perceived her as an intruder. For Célia, she has a kind of 'hyperlove', a devouring love that again has little to do with what Célia might need from her caregiver. Mother wants to be everything for Célia, and she wants Célia to be everything for her. It is a total, intoxicating, voracious love that excludes the external world. The older brother recognises this psychic atmosphere of being devoured by the mother, as he had been in it as well growing up. When Diane decides to go to the grandmother's house, the brother registers something that remains unseen to everyone else: he understands that someone would need to psychically intervene between mother and Célia, caught up in a symbiotic dance choreographed by mother. In other words, he gains access to his traumatically acquired hyper-faculties which allow him to accurately register the psychic danger in which Célia finds herself. In this instance, the brother creates a 'childful' analogy, one that nevertheless aptly and accurately captures the core of the psychic scene. He claims that he will remain at home 'to stop Maman from eating Célia as if she were some coconut cake'. With this, he becomes the saviour, and in a sense sacrifices a part of his own ego to make sure the scene of being smothered by mother's narcissistic love does not repeat itself for Célia.

As I noted above, the Orpha fragment of the psyche brings an account of the emergence of hyper-faculties and over-performance. As a product of the traumatic shock, Orpha operates as 'an unperturbed intelligence which is not restricted by any chronological or spatial resistances in its relation to the environment' (Ferenczi, 1931b, pp. 245–246). In other words, Orpha is connected to acts that might appear clairvoyant. In effect, they are the result of a traumatically enhanced perception. Orpha is capable of registering subtle psychic moves, which can easily be missed by other observers or participants in the scene. Orpha is also able to manifest a special kind of traumatic empathy. This is the result of the many exercises of 'conversion' around which the Orpha fragment of the psyche is organised, where the other is put in the place of a part of the self, and a part of the self is put in the place of the other.

The older brother might manage to 'save' Célia from being completely swallowed by the mother, but this comes at the cost of being trapped in a scene in which a narcissistic caregiver overwhelms the child with an excess of love.

On Orphic Repair

> *As they could not exclude the possibility of a girl, Diane prepared a strategy: she would smother the poor little thing with affection to console her for her mother's coldness. Because it might be too much hope that the unfortunate child would display her older sister's fortitude from the outset. Moreover, the newcomer would have to put up with the*

> *mother's marked preference for her older brother: how could she bear such an injustice.*
>
> (Nothomb, 2017, p. 43; my emphasis)

> *Her heart sank. She was worried for her unfortunate little sister, and, as the car pulled away from their house, she prayed for her, not without also reflecting on the uselessness of her prayers, which had not stopped God from picking the wrong sex for the third child.*
>
> (Nothomb, 2017, p. 45; my emphasis)

We have here a complicated Orphic scene that involves the cold and unavailable mother, the (loved) younger brother, and the (potentially unloved) yet unborn younger sister. The scene is written from the perspective of the older sister, Diane, who already has a younger brother and is confronted with the arrival of a second younger sibling. The protagonist's psyche was traumatically split by the mother's unconscious preference for the younger brother. In the fragment above, this Orphic fragment gains an autonomous functioning, a voice, and performs complex psychic arithmetic: the unborn sibling will not be loved if she is a girl, just like Diane was not loved and was abandoned by the mother. Diane prays so that the unborn child does not have 'the wrong sex'.

Diane thus takes on the task of *Orphic repair*: she imagines that she would be able to love the imagined sister and thus compensate for the mother's lack of love for her girl-children. This is also a scene of a particular kind of Orphic narcissism: the protagonist imagines loving the girlhood of the sister as a way of also being able to love the girlhood within herself. Orpha knows that in this family configuration boys are loved by the mother, while girls are rejected or abandoned. Orpha thus gives a destiny to an overwhelming unconscious communication made by the caregiver (the mother) in relation to what is valuable and worthy of love (the masculinity located in the baby boy is lovable, while the femininity in the baby girl – the protagonist, or other baby girls such as herself – is unlovable).

On Longing for Wholeness

> *Similarly, when she ate the soft-boiled eggs her father was in the habit of making for her, she would eat the white first, saving the delicate yolk for last as she gazes admiringly at it in her plate: this was God, since it*

> *didn't spread. She asked for a spoon, so as not to destroy the miracle, which she placed whole in her mouth.*
>
> (Nothomb, 2017, p. 45)

In this scene the protagonist, Diane, who has known many traumatic splits due to being 'dropped' by her caregivers, is animated by a momentary longing for wholeness, which is expressed in small gestures and her fascination for the 'delicate' yolk of the egg that the father has prepared for her. She is invested in not destroying 'the miracle' of the yolk, in keeping it whole, intact, in its fragile roundness. There is a set of important equivalences here: egg – God – the miracle – wholeness – not spreading. In the midst of fragmentation, eating the miraculous yolk stands for achieving a momentary state of wholeness. It's almost like imitating the wholeness of the egg.

In the consulting room, as they grapple with their states of psychic fragmentation, many analysands have a deep longing for a state of wholeness. This can take many forms and is variably available to conscious elaboration. It is almost as if the patient would like to revert to the state of 'tenderness', to exist in a time *before* the scene of trauma, or before the clash between the language of passion and the language of tenderness. This is perhaps what Ferenczi imaged with the intersection of the 'positive hallucinations' and the 'negative hallucinations' that accompany the process of the identification with the aggressor (Ferenczi, 1933). Through the positive hallucinations, the subject wishes to return to the previous state of tenderness that preceded the trauma. Through the negative hallucinations, the subject creates a psychic position grounded in asserting that 'this is not happening to me'. We can see that this position produces a fundamental alteration of the reality principle: the subject has in their repertoire the denial of overwhelming and unpleasant feelings, often through a combination of negative and positive hallucinations.

The fascinating egg yolk is here a materialised metaphor for this state of longing for wholeness. Diane gets lost in the egg, which stands for God (in the sense of a unifying principle) and for wholeness.

In one of the entries of the *Clinical Diary,* written on 30 July 1932, Ferenczi moves from one of his patient's dreams to dramatising a dialogue between analyst and patient on the theme of psychic wholeness and recollection. Subtly, in this entry, the analyst steps into the position of talking to the *entire* ego of the patient about psychic parts and splits. This is a very interesting analytic posture and direction of analytic address, in which the patient's longing for wholeness is engaged with rather than being left in a hallucinatory state and in the pre-traumatic register. The analyst acknowledges both that the patient is in fragments and that they are longing for wholeness and for recovering the 'lost' parts of the ego. In this dramatised dialogue, the patient asks the analyst,

> why can't I come to terms with the death of the part that has been killed and see that with a great part of my personality I am still alive: why can't I concern myself with the present and the future.

And further along:

> But how are you going to make me suffer the pain that I have skilfully managed to avoid in the trauma without a renewed split, that is, without any repetition of the mental disorder, thereby restoring the unity of my personality, that is, render conscious what has never been conscious before? Does it not seem to you like an impossible undertaking?

Ferenczi here overtly attributes to the patient a conscious longing for wholeness but also a profound doubt that any such state can be achieved. The response of the analyst to the last question is equally interesting, and it relies on some clinical realism, relating to the 'reversibility' of psychic phenomena of splitting: 'My reply: "I don't know myself, but am [convinced] of the reversibility of all psychic processes [...]"'. In other words, what has been split can be linked up or reconnected again.

On Orphic Alliances

> *'I love you, Diane.'*
> *'What's gotten into you?'*
> *'Why aren't you here during the week? I love you so much. I feel better when you are here.'*
> *'Yeah, really.'*
> *'No, it's true. Maman loves me too much, she never leaves me alone.'*

> *'You love it, and you always ask for more.'*
> *'I don't know what to do.'*
> *Diane could sense the truth of her words and she turned to her sister.*
> *'You have to tell her it's not okay.'*
> *'But I love Maman.'*
> *'Of course you do. And that is precisely why you have to tell her, because you love her. You have to tell her she has to leave you alone, that all her kisses are making you sick and she's keeping you from growing up.'*
>
> (Nothomb, 2017, p. 55)

We have here a tragic Orphic dialogue between the older sister and the younger sister. The two children register the mother's state of pathological narcissism and the devouring nature of her love and they are gesturing towards a reparation. We could even think of an 'Orphic alliance' taking place here, where two hyper-perceptive Orphic voices enter into dialogue. In a situation of denial, when the caregivers deny their own seduction and abandonment of the children, the two children construe together a moment of truthfulness. The sense of the veridic that they achieve together is at the core of psychic repair here. The outcome, however, is a tragic one. In the novel, the young sister makes an attempt to convey to the mother her feeling of being suffocated and eaten up by the toxic love. In a striking scene that attests to the functioning of authority, the mother 'breaks' the protesting child into submission again, appealing to her love ('Don't you like my kisses?', asks mother [p.59]), convincing her that she does not actually need more space to breathe and grow and that her protests don't belong to herself but to her jealous older sister. The moment of Orphic alliance is thus very fragile, and it is soon dissolved by the firmer and more resilient forms of infantile obedience. The mother 'moulds' the child out of her own longings and out of her own psychic sense of truth, aligning her again to the mother's narcissistic needs.

Ferenczi does not treat the state of infantile obedience as a given state but as a libidinal puzzle that needs careful consideration. The genealogy of his solution can be found in his 1913 text 'Taming of a Wild Horse', where he offers a minute description of the actions of a 'horse whisperer' who manages a successful domestication of a wild horse. The key of this domestication is neither force and imposition nor mild and gentle seduction but a fast alternation between the two, capable of 'breaking' the animal by causing it an unbearable intensity and the confusion of unmet expectations in terms of the registers of address (from love to dread, in a tight sequence). The tamer seems to make precise tactical use of his knowledge about the effect of this juxtaposition of love and dread, and he first uses affectionate stroking and monotonous lulling talk, followed by authoritative and compelling loud-voice commands. Ferenczi (1913) calls the first tactic 'maternal hypnosis' and the second 'paternal hypnosis'. With this complicated event of submission, the capacity for independent action is lost and so is the capacity for doubt. The subject comes to ignore the validity of their own psychical and physical experience, and delegates judgements to an external force.

On Protective Bladders as Orphic Formations

Listening closely to the voice of Orpha orients us to the creativity of psychic fragments. Indeed, Orphic formations cannot be reduced to a flat present, to omnipotence, triumphalism, and psychic danger. We have seen so far that splitting is more readily available to the psyche than we are used to thinking. I believe we need to continue Ferenczi's project of arranging and systematising images of fragmentation collected from the dreams, hallucinations and fantasies of patients. What does it mean to work with fragments? What do the lives of fragments look like and how might the psychoanalyst be productively involved in these lives?

Taking seriously the instances of radical plasticity of organs and of psychic fragments is also a form of pluralising our life drive imaginary. Organs and body parts are able to reshape themselves or create new configurations. In Ferenczi's *Thalassa*, immersion in the sphere of the life drive takes the form of an investigation into a variety of 'protective' formations that the psycho-soma can create. He looks at various ad hoc protective bladders, vesicles, pustulae filled with fluid, or 'places of abode', usually developed under the strain of the traumatic attack. Such protective creations are directly implicated in psychic survival at the time of catastrophe. There is a complex analogy at play here:

> the supposition that the amniotic fluid represents a sea 'introjected', as it were, into the womb of the mother – a sea in which, as the embryologist

> R. Hertwig says, 'the delicate and easily injured embryo swims and executes movements like a fish in water'.
>
> (Ferenczi, 1924, p. 56)

Ferenczi (1932a) constructs a whole new series of terms that are both clinically and politically interesting: cooperation, conciliation, endurance of suffering, selflessness, appeasement, adaptation to renunciation, self-denial, compromise. In one entry of *The Clinical Diary,* he experiments with a particular modification to the sphere of the dualism death drive/ life drive. He renames them the 'drive of self-assertion' and the 'drive of conciliation'. The 'selflessness' he evokes, including the 'selflessness' of organs, emerges in relation to the scene of trauma. The 'drive for conciliation' appears as a basis of the reality principle. To survive as any sort of individuality means to practice a kind of politics of self-limitation. Ferenczi names this 'the feminine principle' (1924).

It is thus on this backdrop – that of a reconfiguration of the life drive/ death drive dualism – that Ferenczi turns to protective bladders. Protective bladders allow for some partial and hallucinatory integration in a psychic time where the danger of complete disintegration looms. He records that his patient R.N./Elizabeth Severn imagined an expandable bladder formed at the back of her head, where all her pain could accumulate (Ferenczi, 1932a, p. 121). This pain-collecting bladder has a function in surviving the intensity of suffering in the scene of trauma. As Ferenczi writes:

> The patient has the sensation that suddenly, at a painful spot at the back of her head, a bladder is formed, which has room for all her pain. The bladder is almost infinitely expandable. [...] On this painful site on the head [...] an ad hoc bladder is formed, but with this the splitting of personality has begun. A more recent trauma can also overcome the bladder-formation and cause it, so to speak, to burst.
>
> (Ferenczi, 1932a, p. 121)

Ferenczi pays close attention in his clinical work to such odd organs, swelling up and disintegrating, in relation to some detail of the scene. He reflects on the task of the analyst in relation to these Orphic formations. As I mentioned previously, one of these tasks is to reassemble the bladder from its fragments after it bursts or shatters. The bladder-formations often have a key role for the patient connected to psychic survival. Another task is to ensure that the reconstructed bladder is connected with other parts of the ego and thus does not remain isolated.

One of my patients, who suffered extreme physical pain from a very young age, spoke to me about a red box inside her chest where all the pain was deposited. The descriptions of this were very precise: the box had a certain size, texture and intensity of colour. The box would never open, as it condensed decades of intense pain. It would need to stay closed as part of the patient's feeling in a good state of balance. We sometimes talked of the red box, as if circling it in a gentle and interested manner. The red box did not exist in complete isolation from other parts of the ego. It was also not unrepresentable: it came with a series of images, feelings and associations. Still its representation needed to be 'visited' only so often, when one more pain 'item' would need to be deposited there. It would have been a dangerous and ill-advised analytic gesture to try to dissolve the box or seek for it to be entirely integrated with the rest of the ego. The red box is an Orphic formation, and it was needed for surviving extreme pain. It represents a creative psychic solution and I read it mostly as a manifestation of the life drive and the patient's resilience in the face of pain.

Between the Orpha and the Superego

To the three Freudian 'agencies' or 'systems' of the psyche – id, ego, and superego – Ferenczi has added a fourth one, Orpha. The question of how the systems relate to one another is a fascinating one. In the clinic, we often wonder how the system of the superego relates to the system of the ego, for instance. This relationship can be punitive or cruel. The inter-systemic relations between the superego and the Orpha, or the ego and the Orpha, represent as yet uncharted territory.

In brief, in Ferenczi's work we can come to imagine and work clinically with a superego that is itself internally fragmented. Various parts of the superego have distinct relations with other Ferenczian agencies or psychic fragments. Through an image of a fragmented superego, we can also recover the fundamental paradox that Freud inscribed into the superego and which was 'diluted' after Freud by an emphasis placed on the prohibitive aspect of the superego. The superego is thus the inheritor of a paradoxical injunction: 'you must be like father' and 'you cannot be like father' are the two facets of this injunction, which the ego has the impossible task to respond to. The superego cannot therefore be accurately described as an 'agency of prohibition' but as a paradoxical agency.

When this paradox creates very loud effects of psychic suffering, the 'cruel superego' can find itself acting in conjunction with Orpha. In a sense, the cruel superego knows how to mobilise Orpha for its own sadomasochistic purposes, making the 'life' of the ego impossible.

As we noted, Orpha does not operate with any spatio-temporal limitations. It is triumphant: it results from a scene of survival in improbable circumstances. This means that Orpha omnipotence 'sounds' very different in the consulting room to superego omnipotence. The omnipotence of the superego speaks in the voice of 'you must do more, you must do better, you must be more like your father, while you cannot be like your father'. The omnipotence of Orpha speaks in a different voice: 'let's see if you can pass this test, if you can achieve this, right now', or 'you can be anything, anytime, your powers are unlimited'. We have seen above that Orpha operates in an eternal present, an imperative, cruel, glamorous present. There is no possibility of historical depth here, or a sense of being inscribed in a line of inheritance, or even of the temporality of the *Nachträglichkeit*; there is just a single flat surface of an all-engulfing present which contains all the acts.

The complex functioning in conjunction of Orpha and the superego can create a parallel, traumatically derived, 'fake' reality testing: it is like a mirage, a cunning seduction, exposing the subject to great and often deadly risks. The subject is seduced into believing that the risks undertaken are in the name of 'survival', an ancient territory of Orpha. The alliance between Orpha and the cruel superego is a tragic one, and it generates a 'private morality' that has to do with the details of the trauma scene and not with observing the world out there, or with observing the other, or the self in relation to the other. The psychic atmosphere here is one of many imperatives that transform small, mundane, insignificant experiences into colossal, exquisite, insurmountable tasks.

On Reconstruction

If the psyche presents itself as a kind of mosaic of parts, some of which are alive and some of which are deadened (de-libidinised), then what does it mean to say that some form of post-catastrophic reconstruction is possible, and what does such a reconstruction rest upon? In his *Clinical Diary*, Ferenczi (1932a, p. 176) makes an intriguing note: 'in a manner which to us appears mystical, the ego fragments remain linked to one another, however distorted and hidden this may be'. I believe this note is a metapsychological assumption rather than a metaphorical statement. This is confirmed by the fact that the 'link' preserved between the split parts of the psyche also makes its apparition in dreams and dream-like images and states. Patients sometimes bring us dreams of a cut-off body part that is still connected by one thread to the body. In one of the sections above, we analysed a dream of fragments of patient R.N., as it was recorded in the *Clinical Diary.* This dream contained an imagery of threads and their collapse, such as that of an interrupted long-distance telephone call. In such dream imagery, what is significant is not only the severed organ/head but also the *thread* that connects it to the body.

If we take this proposition seriously, what emerges as a question is: where and how can this thread be found and in which way can it be used for the psychoanalytic process? In the consulting room, this question brings us to the crucial importance of *regression* for the healing of trauma. The clinician will know that as a result of a traumatic shock, one part of the personality can 'die' (or, in other words, the libido can fully withdraw from a part of the personality), while the part that survives the trauma can wake up from the shock with 'a gap in memory' (or, to be more precise, with a gap in conscious memory or the system of memory of the ego). The 'thread' that we are discussing passes through the system of memory of the id which has an entirely different inscription mechanism from the system of memory of the ego. This does not mean that nothing was ever presented or preserved in the unconscious, but that to be able to access it, a re-enactment by way of regression is needed. Ferenczi (1931a, p. 140) noted that often in the second part of the analytic cure, what the patient experiences is a 'collapse of the intellectual superstructure', accompanied by a 'breaking through of the fundamental situation, which after all is always primitive and strongly affective in character'.

This kind of regression will make possible a 'new beginning' – a term that Michael Bálint (1968) will later put at the centre of his propositions on 'benign regression' and 'the basic fault'. What is repeated in this state of regression is the original conflict between the ego and the environment, as well as the painful intrapsychic solutions found for this conflict, in search of fresh and better resolution.

Homo Infans

We have seen thus far that Ferenczi constructs a revised metapsychology. We have approached it mostly through its *clinical* implications: through what it shifts in the psychoanalytic dispositif, in the transference, in the way we image the relationships between psychic agencies for each patient. But the clinic is a deeply *political* place, and the way we envision the territories and processes of the mind goes hand in hand with what kind of social or political worlds we deem possible. Let us consider here one figure in Ferenczi's work – sometimes enigmatic, sometimes theoretically dense, sometimes philosophically invested: *the figure of the child*. It would perhaps be more accurate to speak of Ferenczi's 'children', as there are different hypostases of the child that populate his world. Firstly, there is the actual child, the one who suffers the trauma and enters the triangle of the confusion of tongues. This child makes herself present in the consulting room, in the analysis of the adult (Ferenczi, 1931a), in the process of repeating the infantile trauma, in the presence of the analyst. The analysis itself proceeds as the interaction of two children playing (Ferenczi, 1933). By this, Ferenczi means that for the analysis to be successful, the analyst needs to be able to make herself vulnerable, to exit an authoritative position, and to have gained access to the childful, traumatised part of her own self. Secondly, there is the 'wise baby' – a psychoanalytic construction we have examined above and that has come to stand for the split subject that resulted from the trauma. Thirdly, there is Orpha – a fragment of the psyche, formed in the process of splitting, which also acquires qualities of a true, novel psychic agency. Fourthly, there is *homo infans*, a philosophical construction at the centre of Ferenczi's utopian ideas – his idea of the emancipated subject.

This intriguing plurality of images of the child opens a window onto the various dimensions of Ferenczi's work. Ferenc Erős (2014) comments on the various ways in which we can read Ferenczi's *Clinical Diary*: as a metaphysical treatise on the relation between body and soul, passion and reason; as an essay on moral philosophy, grounding a psychoanalytically informed ethic; as a politico-philosophical essay. Antal Bókay (2015) alerts us to the child functioning in Ferenczi's work as a philosophical-anthropological category. Bókay (2015, p. 49) suggests it is no accident that, in Ferenczi's writings, the child [*Kind*] appears in the singular, while the adults [*Erwachsenen*] appear in the plural. This is the case as well in his famous 1933 paper, 'The Confusion of Tongues Between Adults and the Child' (Ferenczi, 1933).

In the last decade of his life, Ferenczi developed the conviction that we are all 'wise babies' to some extent and that a certain amount of splitting is inescapable, irrespective of how much love and care we receive from our environment and primary objects. There is a certain traumatic autonomisation of faculties (sometimes even a production of 'new organs') that needs to be relived in the analytic frame.

Ferenczi's most political ideas on radical mutuality are also constructed around the image of the child. In the *Clinical Diary*, in the context of a discussion on sublimation, Ferenczi talks about a 'mutual goodwill' which is 'more primary, natural, nonneurotic' (Ferenczi, 1932a, p. 151). If we are able to imagine a child who has not been subjected to traumatic suffering, then we can also imagine that she can share pleasures with the environment and even take pleasure, without feelings of envy, in the expansion of this environment. Secondly, we can imagine the suppression of hate impulses, ending the 'chains of acts of cruelties' which appear to us like 'blood feuds' (ibid, p. 146). Thirdly, the scope of human action is imagined as greatly extended, as humans would experience 'the contact of an individual with the whole universe' (ibid). Fourthly, radical mutuality finds expression in a particular human version of adaptation to life in common: 'Higher (also ethical) human knowledge is a *return to compromise* – or the principle of *appeasement*, which exists everywhere' (ibid, p. 153). Ferenczi's child is thus not the legacy-child, the family-bound child, the blood-child, the child-to-be-educated – a projection screen for our domesticated hopes of the future or an ideological image for constructing the nation. It is a more enigmatic and radical figure: more like the parentless, playful survivor of extraordinary violence who has gained access to a plurality of complicated temporalities.

In one of his notes, 'The Two Extremes: Credulity and Scepticism', Ferenczi speaks of 'psychognosis' or 'gnosis' which he defines as 'the hope that it is possible, through an adequate profound relaxation, to gain access to a direct path to a past experience, which can be accepted without any other interpretation as being true' (Ferenczi, 1932b, p. 263). This is not in the least a nostalgic move, a longing for an innocent, perfect, unspoilt childhood. Instead, in a similar way to Walter Benjamin, Ferenczi has a kind of epistemology attached to his turning towards the past. The value is not in immersion or dwelling in the past but precisely in the act of *veering towards the past* that we as subjects perform. What is to be achieved through 'psychognosis' is not a direct access to the experience 'of how things truly were' but an *effect of authenticity* and an *effect of veracity*. Utopia is, here, the multiplication and expansion of such psychic effects of authenticity. The post-traumatic state is thus, paradoxically, fuller in possibilities for enrichment and more radically relational than the pre-traumatic state.

The multiplication of the effects of authenticity brought by psychognosis can approximate a state of clairvoyance. This clairvoyance is not some mystical construct but a result of the relationship with the past. As Ferenczi writes:

> It is impossible to foresee what the consequences would be for knowledge if people were freed from this anxiety and dared to examine and recognise the world in its own quite self-evident form; how much further that could lead, than even the most audacious of what nowadays we call phantasies. Really mastering anxiety, or rather overcoming it, might perhaps make us quite clairvoyant, and might help humanity to solve apparently insoluble problems.
>
> (Ferenczi, 1932a, pp. 129–130)

Ferenczi is interested in this kind of clairvoyance to the extent that it can enrich collective life. 'For the visionary adult', Ferenczi writes, 'the infantile amnesia disappears, and, due to the lifting of the barriers of repression, he is able to establish communication with the visionary child, and the capacities of the latter stay with the adult' (ibid).

In two short manuscripts, 'Parallel between Marxism, Communism and Anarchism', and 'Parallel between Psychoanalysis and Liberal Socialism', which we have access to through Ferenc Erős's translation (2014), Ferenczi introduces his political actor: *homo infans*. He writes, somewhat enigmatically: '*Homo infans* is "basic structure", but *homo oeconomicus* is already "superstructure"' (Ferenczi, cited in Erős, 2014). Here is a succinct dialogue with Marxian theory, but one which gives us clues as to the tremendous place that *homo infans* occupies. So how might we think of *homo infans*? *Homo infans* is the political transformation of Orpha. Perhaps a subject who acts *by* childhood, a subject who has accepted their libidinal constitution of 'wise baby' and has touched the Orpha fragment of their psyche. Perhaps a subject who has achieved an effect of authenticity in relation to the wounded child within the psyche, the split child, the child that has suffered the intrusion of the language of passion. Perhaps a subject who knows both what polysemy looks like and what happens when it is interrupted and words become heavy and nearly material. Perhaps a subject who no longer needs to deny their erotic constitution.

References

Bálint, M. (1968). *The Basic Fault. Therapeutic Aspects of Regression*. London: Tavistock.

Bókay, A. (2015). The child as a traumatic self-component in Ferenczi's later psychoanalysis. *American Journal of Psychoanalysis*, 75(1): 46–56.

Bonomi, C. (2018). *The Cut and the Building of Psychoanalysis, Vol. 2: Sigmund Freud and Sándor Ferenczi*. London & New York, NY: Routledge.

Erős, F. (2014). Freedom and authority in the *Clinical Diary*. *American Journal of Psychoanalysis*, 74(4): 367–380.

Ferenczi, S. (1913). Taming of a wild horse. In: *Final Contributions to the Problems and Methods of Psycho-analysis* (transl. by E. Mosbacher, pp. 336–340). London: Karnac, 1994.

Ferenczi, S. (1920). Psycho-analytical observations on tic. In: *Further Contributions to the Theory and Technique of Psycho-analysis* (transl. by J. I. Suttie, pp. 142–174). London: Karnac, 1994.

Ferenczi, S. (1923). The dream of the 'clever baby'. In: *Further Contributions to the Theory and Technique of Psycho-analysis* (transl. by J. I. Suttie, pp. 349–350). London: Karnac, 1994.

Ferenczi, S. (1924). *Thalassa. A Theory of Genitality* (transl. by H. A. Bunker). London & New York, NY: Karnac, 1989.

Ferenczi, S. (1926a). The problem of acceptance of unpleasant ideas – advances in knowledge of the sense of reality. In: *Further Contributions to the Theory and Technique of Psycho-analysis* (transl. by J. I. Suttie, pp. 366–379). London: Karnac, 1994.

Ferenczi, S. (1926b). Organ neuroses and their treatment. In: *Final Contributions to the Problems and Methods of Psycho-Analysis* (transl. by E. Mosbacher, pp. 22–28). London: Karnac, 1994.

Ferenczi, S. (1929). The unwelcome child and his death instinct. In: *Final Contributions to the Problems and Methods of Psycho-analysis* (transl. by E. Mosbacher, pp. 102–107). London: Karnac, 1994.

Ferenczi, S. (1930a). Autoplastic and alloplastic adaptation. In: *Final Contributions to the Problems and Methods of Psycho-analysis* (transl. by E. Mosbacher, p. 221). London: Karnac, 1994.

Ferenczi, S. (1930b). On the analytic construction of mental mechanism. In: *Final Contributions to the Problems and Methods of Psycho-Analysis* (transl. by E. Mosbacher, p. 222). London: Karnac, 1994.

Ferenczi, S. (1930c). Trauma and striving for health. In: *Final Contributions to the Problems and Methods of Psycho-analysis* (transl. by E. Mosbacher, pp. 230–231). London: Karnac, 1994.

Ferenczi, S. (1931a). Child-analysis in the analysis of adults. In: *Final Contributions to the Problems and Methods of Psycho-analysis* (transl. by E. Mosbacher, pp. 126–142). London: Karnac, 1994.

Ferenczi, S. (1931b). The birth of intellect. In: *Final Contributions to the Problems and Methods of Psycho-analysis* (transl. by E. Mosbacher, pp. 244–246). London: Karnac, 1994.

Ferenczi, S. (1931c). Trauma and anxiety. In: *Final Contributions to the Problems and Methods of Psycho-analysis* (transl. by E. Mosbacher, p. 249–250). London: Karnac, 1994.

Ferenczi, S. (1932a). *The Clinical Diary of Sándor Ferenczi*, ed. by J. Dupont (transl. by M. Bálint & N. Z. Jackson). Cambridge, MA: Harvard University Press, 1995.
Ferenczi, S. (1932b). The two extremes: Credulity and scepticism. In: *Final Contributions to the Problems and Methods of Psycho-analysis* (transl. by E. Mosbacher, pp. 263–264). London: Karnac, 1994.
Ferenczi, S. (1933). The confusion of tongues between adults and the child. In: *Final Contributions to the Problems and Methods of Psycho-analysis* (transl. by E. Mosbacher, pp. 156–167). London: Karnac, 1994.
Fortune, C. (1993). Sándor Ferenczi's analysis of 'RN': A critically important case in the history of psychoanalysis. *British Journal of Psychotherapy*, 9(4): 436–443.
Graves, R. (1992). *The Greek Myths, Complete Edition.* New York, NY: Penguin Books.
Green, A. (1996). *On Private Madness.* London: Karnac.
Harris, A. (2015). 'Language is there to bewilder itself and others': Theoretical and clinical contributions of Sabina Spielrein. *Journal of the American Psychoanalytic Association*, 63(4): 727–767.
Hristeva, G. (2013). 'Uterus loquitur': Trauma and the human organism in Ferenczi's 'physiology of pleasure'. *American Journal of Psychoanalysis*, 73(4): 339–352.
Hristeva, G. (2019). 'Primordial Chant'. Sándor Ferenczi as an Orphic Poet. *The American Journal of Psychoanalysis*, 79(4): 517–539.
Kerényi, K. (1959). *The Heroes of the Greeks*. London: Thames and Hudson.
Nothomb, A. (2000). *The Character of Rain* (transl. by T. Bent). London: Faber and Faber.
Nothomb, A. (2017). *Strike Your Heart* (transl. by A. Anderson). New York, NY: Europa Editions, 2018.
Rachman, A. (2017). *Elizabeth Severn: The 'Evil Genius' of Psychoanalysis*. London: Routledge.
Rudnytsky, P. L. (2017). The other side of the story: Severn on Ferenczi and mutual analysis. In: E. Severn (ed.), *The Discovery of the Self: A Study in Psychological Cure*. London: Routledge.
Rudnytsky, P. L. (2021). *Mutual Analysis: Ferenczi, Severn, and the Origins of Trauma Theory*. Abingdon & New York, NY: Routledge.
Severn, E. (1933). *The Discovery of the Self: A Study in Psychological Cure*. London: Routledge, 2017.
Smith, N. A. (1998). 'Orpha reviving': Toward an honorable recognition of Elizabeth Severn. *International Forum of Psychoanalysis*, 7(4): 241–246.
Smith, N. A. (1999). From Oedipus to Orpha: Revisiting Ferenczi and Severn's landmark case. *American Journal of Psychoanalysis*, 59(4): 345–366.
Soreanu, R. (2023a). Catastrophe and the creativity of fragments: Toward a phenomenology of the scene of trauma. In: R. Soreanu, J. Staberg, & J. Willner (eds), *Ferenczi Dialogues: On Trauma and Catastrophe* (pp. 145–192). Leuven: Leuven University Press.
Soreanu, R. (2018b). *Working-Through Collective Wounds: Trauma, Denial, Recognition in the Brazilian Uprising.* London: Palgrave Macmillan.
Spielrein, S. (1912). Destruction as the cause of coming into being. *Journal of Analytical Psychology*, 39(2): 155–186, 1994.
Stanton, M. (1991). *Sándor Ferenczi: Reconsidering Active Intervention*. London: Free Association Books.
Wilson, E. A. (2015). *Gut Feminism*. Durham, NC: Duke University Press.
Wolstein, B. (1992). Resistance interlocked with countertransference: RN and Ferenczi, and American interpersonal relations. *Contemporary Psychoanalysis*, 28(1): 172–190.

Chapter 4

The Analyst's Times

Time and Psychoanalysis

Time contains infinite worlds. As Gilles Deleuze (1988) stated, it is 'a polyphony of polyphonies'. In this chapter, I explore ideas of time in the work of Sándor Ferenczi with the aim of clarifying and furthering his 'metapsychology of the analyst's mental process during analysis' (Ferenczi, 1928, p. 98). In other words, I talk about the psychoanalyst's times. Ideas of time in the psychoanalytic process function as *meta-constructions*: they organise the scene. As the word suggests, I derive the term from Freud's 'constructions in analysis' (1937). Meta-constructions are the grids within which analysts, like archaeologists, place other constructions during the analytic session. In the case of time, such grids have two aspects: an artisanal one, through which the analyst works time into specific sessions, and a theoretical one, through which the analyst elucidates the idea of time on which the sessions rest. As Jacob Arlow wrote, '[h]ardly any other profession functions in as intimate and consistent an involvement with time as does psychoanalysis. Considerations of time figure prominently in every aspect of our work' (1986, p. 507).

In recent decades, several psychoanalytic voices have offered important reflections on temporality and analysis (see Hartocollis, 1972, 1974, 1983, 2003; Arlow, 1984, 1986; Sabbadini, 1989, 2014; Laget, 1995; Perelberg, 2008; Cabré, 2008; Birksted-Breen, 2012). André Green (2000, 2009) spoke strongly, however, about the distorting operations that time has lately suffered in psychoanalytic theory.[1] To address what Green specifically referred to as the 'ignorance of time', the 'murder of time', and the 'misrecognition of temporality' (2009, p. 16), this chapter turns to Ferenczi's writings that acknowledge the importance and complexity of temporality for the analyst's process. In his works, time is neither ignored, nor murdered, nor

DOI: 10.4324/9781032715926-5

misrecognised; instead, it is woven into a pluralistic meta-construction. His writings avoid the psychoanalytic fascination with the idea of timelessness that arises from a consideration of the atemporal aspects of the psyche and the atemporal nature of the drive. Captivated by this 'timeless time' and by the 'timelessness of the unconscious', one can miss the qualitatively different threads of time that organise the psychoanalytic encounter.

Ferenczi's contributions to psychoanalytic technique have variously been discussed by reference to notions of active technique, elasticity, mutuality, and tact. What holds these contributions together, however, is precisely Ferenczi's unique approach to time and, in particular, his capacity to consider the mythological, historical, and intersubjective dimensions of time. In what follows, and in a search for a good enough metaphor, I identify three threads of time: a tangent, a segment, and a meandering line. Each corresponds to a Ferenczian time: originary time, organic time, and pulsating time. I bring a clinical vignette to capture the different threads of time in the consulting room, and I then discuss the implications of this plurality of times for the position of the analyst.

First Thread: Originary Time or the Tangent-out

Ferenczi's originary time is his most daring but also his most obscure dimension of time. Its opacity grows out of the very history of psychoanalysis; in particular, it grows out of early efforts at demarcating psychoanalysis from occultism and spiritualism, and at institutionalising it as a science. In his 1933 obituary of Ferenczi, the English psychoanalyst and psychical researcher John Rickman described him as 'one of the most adventurous speculative researchers' of the Society of Psychical Research, of which they both had been members (Rickman, 1933, p. 124). Indeed, Ferenczi had tried out automatic writing; he had organised telepathy experiments with Frau Seidler, a Berlin divinatory, and with Frau Jelinek, a Hungarian somnambulist (Gyimesi, 2012); and he had followed closely for eight years the mystical investigations of Elizabeth Severn, a patient with whom he developed his ideas on mutuality. One of his first publications, an essay on spiritism, carries an uninhibited expression of his early pluralistic disposition. Ferenczi writes:

> In the present state of our culture most of the educated imbibe in school the principles of atomic materialism. The world consists of an infinite

> mass of indivisible particles of various sizes whose vibrations produce light, warmth, electricity, and so forth. Consciousness itself is a product of masses of brain material. Our physics instructor found it easy to talk of all this with full conviction. From his point of view everything was very simple. There were 60–70 different atoms (since then we have 10 more), 8–10 different kinds of other vibrations; this was the essence of the universe. He who spoke of uniexistence, soul or metaphysics was a fool.
>
> (Ferenczi, 1899, p. 140)

Material classifications and the scientism of his era left Ferenczi unconvinced and quite curious about exploring 'uniexistence' even before encountering Freud and Freudian psychoanalysis. It is important to note that Ferenczi was not a monist but a pluralist, as he believed that there are different strata of reality, each of them with their own properties and ontologies. Later, his interest in telepathy and thought transference filtered through the scientific project of psychoanalysis.

Ferenczi, not without enthusiasm, shared with Freud that he had established a series of connections between telepathy and transference. As he playfully wrote to Freud on 22 November 1910, on his next visit to Vienna he would introduce himself as 'court astrologer of the psychoanalysts' (Freud et al., 1993, pp. 235–236). In his response the following month, Freud explicitly asked him to postpone the publication of his conclusions for three years.[2] In fact, Ferenczi never published his thoughts on telepathy from that period. Throughout the years, he remained reserved in elucidating the relationship between telepathic thought transference (*Gedankenübertragung*), intergenerational transmission (*Übertragung*), and transference (*Übertragung*). He carefully veiled the way he incorporated into psychoanalytic technique what Stephen Frosh (2012) calls the 'horizontal dimension' of psychic transmission (what travels consciously or unconsciously from one person to another) and the 'vertical dimension' of psychic transmission (what travels from one time period or generation to another). In his *Clinical Diary*, Ferenczi writes:

> It is possible that here we are facing a fourth 'narcissistic wound' namely that even the intelligence of which we are so proud, though analysts, is not our property but must be replaced or regenerated through

> the *rhythmic outpouring of the ego into the universe*, which alone is all knowing and therefore intelligent. But more of this another time.
>
> (Ferenczi, 1932, p. 33, emphasis added)

This fragment was written in Ferenczi's last year of life and little opportunity remained to elucidate this striking proposition. The pluralistic and non-materialistic traces of his thought led up to 'the rhythmic outpouring of the ego into the universe'.

Ferenczi's *Thalassa* (1924), in which he developed a series of ontogenetic–phylogenetic analogies, marked his most adventurous experiment with originary time. Only through analogy, not through chronology, could one grasp originary time. It could not even be elucidated as regression from present to past. Instead, originary time appeared as a tangent of the lived present. This tangent-out might be imagined as a line of highly accelerated travel touching two temporal periods in which two series of elements stand in similar relations to one another. Analogical thinking meant sustaining contact with *both* series of elements, as a tangent touches on two circles.

As Deleuze (1985) argues, originary time must be understood as the most complicated state. Chiefly due to its undifferentiation, it is not broken apart or developed into a series of dimensions, but rather falls back to the birth of the world (see Pelbart, 2010, p. 10). In *Thalassa*, the tangent crosses between the 'intrauterine existence of higher mammals' and their 'aboriginal piscine period' in which the 'relations' of the elements to each other are marked by *post-catastrophic emergence* (1924, p. 45). For Ferenczi, adaptation and creativity were post-catastrophic events, or as he explained: 'birth itself [is] nothing but a recapitulation on the part of the individual of the great catastrophe which at the time of the recession of the ocean forced so many animals, and certainly our own animal ancestors, to adapt themselves to land existence' (Ferenczi, 1924, p. 45). Moving between ontogenesis and phylogenesis, Ferenczi elucidates elements in the series of post-catastrophic emergence:

> The possession of an organ of copulation, the development within the maternal womb, and the circumvention of the great danger of desiccation—these three thus form an indestructible biological unity which must constitute the ultimate basis of the symbolic identity of the womb

> with the sea and the earth on the one hand, and of the male member with the child and the fish on the other.
>
> (Ferenczi, 1924, p. 50)

Ferenczi's analogical thinking differs from the Saussurean division of the sign into the material signifier (the word) and the conceptual signified (the thing referred to by the sound). For Ferenczi, things have meaning in their immediate materiality. Meaning is not detached, abstracted, or located elsewhere. Materiality is not a lower order that entraps us while semantic fullness remains the horizon towards which we aspire: 'the symbol—a thing of flesh and blood', he writes in a 1921 essay, perhaps with the ink of a poet (Ferenczi, 1921a, p. 352). Here Ferenczi's analogical thinking shares ground with Félix Guattari's semiotics. Guattari writes:

> There is no language in itself. What specifies human language is precisely that it never refers back to itself, it always remains open to all other modes of semiotization.
>
> (Guattari, 2011, p. 27)

Ferenczian semiotics differentiates unsubstantial allegory from the symbol (Ferenczi, 1913, p. 280). Not every analogy is symbolic in a psychoanalytic sense. First, it has a physiological basis; it 'expresses in some ways the whole body or its functions' (Ferenczi, 1921a, p. 355). Second, one of the two terms of an analogy that can be considered symbolic – a thing, an idea – is invested in consciousness with inexplicable, overcharged affect. This surplus of affect derives from unconscious identification with another thing or idea to which it actually belongs. This analogical thinking allows Ferenczi in *Thalassa* to move quite freely from smaller to greater catastrophes and to draw a tangent to originary times.

When Ferenczi distinguishes between unsubstantial analogy and symbolic analogy, he contrasts the two-dimensionality of the former with the three-dimensionality of the latter. What comprises the third dimension? It is the analogical trip that the mind/body of the analyst takes to connect two series of elements that bear a homology, where one series is invested with overcharged affect. Where the split between two areas of the psyche was – or where the split between the body and the mind was – a tangent of elucidation is drawn and with it a new subject emerges, one capable of sustaining the experience of the symbol as a thing of flesh and blood.

Ferenczi's notes on analogical thinking bring us to complications around the analyst's plural being in time. Those complications prevent us from reducing the analyst's mentality to a timelessness in which the attention fluctuates in reverie, beyond the demands of Kronos. Thomas Ogden (1997) describes conscious reverie as one of the analyst's mental states during a session. He recognises its roles in the elucidation of the unconscious experience of the patient, as he explains:

> 'Reverie is a principal form of re-presentation of the unconscious (largely intersubjective) experience of analyst and analysand. The analytic use of reverie is the process by which unconscious experience is made into verbally symbolic metaphors that re-present unconscious aspects of ourselves to ourselves'.
>
> (Ogden, 1997, p. 727)

But Ferenczi would here object to the centrality of linguistic symbols. Words, too, can be bound to unsubstantial allegory, just as things can comprise the heart of symbols.

Similarly, Ferenczi's tangential temporality cannot be equated with enigmatic regression to originary times. César Botella and Sára Botella (2005), for example, describe through the notion of 'figurability' a state of mind in the analyst akin to the night dream. Figurability is predicated on 'the existence of a capacity of the psyche to create a sensorial quality from a singular and complex unconscious process' (Botella & Botella, 2005, p. 10). The analyst, they argue, must allow for a state of 'formal regression' (Botella & Botella, 2005, p. 47), as floating attention no longer suffices to access what lies beyond the mnemic trace. A Ferenczian figurability, however, would not merely fluctuate or reach backwards to the past but would manage to touch upon two temporalities at once, keeping that double contact while elucidating the overcharge of affect in one of them.[3]

Bion's metaphorical image of suspended, unfocused attention, paradoxically both effortless and purposeful, resonates with Ferenczi's analogical thought. Bion describes this mental state as 'a positive act of refraining from both memory and desire' (Bion, 1970, p. 31). Ferenczi's analogical thinking – his own positive act of reframing – is, however, sharper. It is expressed in the grammar: this set of relations in this temporality is akin to the other set of relations in the other temporality. This grammar lies at the core of symbolisation. Such verbalised metaphors or symbols work in the session as a true 'third object' (Winnicott, 1971; Benjamin, 1988) between the analyst and the analysand, creating, in Birksted-Breen's words, 'an "other" or "otherness" that does not produce intolerable jealousy' (Birksted-Breen, 2012, p. 827) and that allows a 're-libidinalisation of the analysis' (Birksted-Breen, 2012, p. 828). In this way, analogical thinking creates an internal thirdness within the analyst as well, where both interpretive work and theoretical elaboration can take place.

There remains, of course, an omnipresent possibility of interruption. Keeping to Ferenczi's account of the symbolic, we can always slip in and out of our words, or we can stumble over our things. The genesis of these interruptions is in the originary catastrophe itself, which can reverberate in smaller catastrophes. It is worth noting that, unlike Lacan's 'coups' (1988), the analyst does not orchestrate these interruptions merely to produce interpretative results for the patient. Instead, the interruptions reflect the internal experience of the analyst who is unafraid of slipping or stumbling. In the process of being interrupted, something very particular happens for Ferenczi: we enter a type of post-catastrophic mode that is more prone to creativity. To keep to our metaphor, an interrupted tangent becomes open for symbolisation and elucidates the two terms of an analogy in a fuller way.

Second Thread: Organic Time or the Segment

Segmentation, or sequence, defines Ferenczi's second temporal thread. It acknowledges the finite nature of psychoanalytic process: not only must every analysis end, but also each analysis must limit itself to the shortest time that can be productive for the patient (see Arlow, 1986; Hartocollis, 2003; Sabbadini, 1989). Further, not only is the finitude of the psychoanalytic treatment at issue but so is the finitude of the analyst and the analysand. What emerges from a series of Ferenczian writings on technique is a sense of self-limitation, one that flows from observing the phases of an organism's birth, maturation, and death. This temporal disposition I call organic time.

An affinity exists between Ferenczi's organic time and the idea of progressive development in the English school of psychoanalysis. As we see in Winnicott, emotional development occurs in successive phases. As such, the temporality of analysis becomes one of delayed action, of waiting, of continuous duration. Ferenczi, however, places emphasis on segmentation, on breaking apart the treatment into elemental phases and locating oneself in its unfolding, from the beginning of the cure to its final stages. But Ferenczi does not confine himself to noting the beginning, middle, and end; he posits a phased theory of transference and countertransference and classifies the analyst's mental actions in each segment. In Ferenczi's words, this amounts to a 'metapsychology of the analyst's mental process during analysis' (Ferenczi, 1928, p. 98). Transference and countertransference divide into different phases, each linked with a series of anticipations on the part of the analyst. This sense of organicity is a manifestation of libido, both of the analysand and the analyst, and Ferenczi produces a true laboratory for discerning the movements of both libidos during the separate phases of the analytic process.

In 'On the Technique of Psychoanalysis', Ferenczi (1919) leads us through the phases of countertransference. Using the image of a 'honeymoon of the analysis', he argues that in the first phase:

> one is miles from considering, let alone mastering, the counter-transference. One yields to every affect that the doctor-patient relationship might evoke, is moved by the patient's sad experiences, probably, too, by his phantasies, and is indignant with all those who wish him ill. In a word, one makes all their interests one's own.
>
> (Ferenczi, 1919, p. 187)

This stage – marked by strong manifestations of empathy – can seldom lead to major analytic advances; it merely prepares the ground. In the second phase – labelled 'the resistance against the counter-transference' – the analyst, after painfully learning the countertransference symptoms, risks becoming 'too abrupt and repellent towards the patient; this would retard the appearance of the transference, the pre-condition of every successful psychoanalysis' (Ferenczi, 1919, p. 188). The third segment or phase, 'the control of counter-transference', is a hybrid time, both mythical and organic. It is, so to speak, a time segment that breaks out of itself. Here the freely moving libido of the analyst is the main tool of work. As Ferenczi writes: 'This constant oscillation between the free play of phantasy and critical scrutiny presupposes freedom and uninhibited motility of psychic excitation on the doctor's part, however, that can hardly ever be demanded in another sphere' (Ferenczi, 1919, p. 189). In the last phase of analysis, the successful mirror of the analyst's uninhibited motility will be the 'weaning of the libido' (Ferenczi & Rank, 1925, p. 12). In this phase, the patient shows the ability to withdraw libido from the analysis and redirect it outward.

Through attention to segmented time, Ferenczi opens the way to acknowledging a striking inversion: sometimes countertransference precedes transference. Analysts, who are considered throughout the entire *Clinical Diary* as part of a 'structure to be erected by two parties' (Haynal, 1999, p. 318), bring their own transferences that run with, not counter to, the analytic process. The analyst's time is less silent and self-effacing than we are accustomed to believe; analysis is not a time-free container guiding the patient into the timelessness of the unconscious. It is time-bound in a way that allows the emergence of a horizontal dimension. The analyst and the analysand occupy the same ontological stratum, producing, in the words of the *Clinical Diary*, 'the impression of two equally terrified children who compare their experiences, and because of their common fate understand each other completely and instinctively try to comfort each other' (Ferenczi, 1932, p. 56). This common time allows for a horizontal therapeutic alliance in which the analyst is not fixed in the place of the father or mother but travels to the places that the cure demands. But while still emphasising this alliance, Ferenczi also ascribes differentiated roles to the analyst and analysand. As he argues, the situation of the analyst is similar in many respects to that of the midwife, who as far as possible attempts to remain a mere observer of a natural process until required at critical moments to intervene and aid a birth that is not progressing spontaneously. In his role, the analyst makes an empathic intervention into organic time.

Ferenczi acknowledges that moving forward and backward through segments of time requires an anchor in the present, a 'here-and-now' technique. He and Otto Rank explain this in *The Development of Psychoanalysis*:

> The analyst must take into account that almost every expression of his patient springs from several periods, but he must give his chief attention to the present reaction. Only from this point of view he can succeed in uncovering the roots of the actual reaction in the past, which means changing the attempts of the patient to repeat into remembering. In this process he need pay little attention to the future. One may quietly leave this care to the person himself who has been sufficiently enlightened about his past and present mental strivings. The historic, cultural and

> phylogenetic analogies also need, in the most part, not be discussed in the analysis. The patient need hardly ever, and the analyst extremely seldom, occupy himself with this early period.
>
> (Ferenczi & Rank, 1925, p. 38)

This passage describes austere self-containment within the present; organic time forms the analyst's horizon of self-restraint. Reflection on historical, cultural, and phylogenetic analogies – on originary time – remains fundamentally a solitary act not shared with the patient in any direct form. Again, the psychoanalyst looks at psychic life just as the midwife observes a natural birth. Here the main operations in the economy of the analyst's mind are segmentation, sequencing, and thinking through phases.

Segments drawn in the mind help to anchor the analyst's temporal metaconstruction. Stated another way, the discipline required to make sense of transference and to break time apart – in the first instance, in the second instance, in the last instance – combats the illusion of timelessness. We thus find in Ferenczi the first psychoanalyst to voice a phased theory of countertransference and to make consciousness of organic life a vehicle of self-limitation and technical clarification.

Third Thread: Pulsating Time or the Meandering Line

The third thread of time – which I represent as a meandering line – leads to Ferenczi's theory of countertransference. This is a time of pulsations, when the analyst becomes attuned to what Ferenczi, in 'The Elasticity of Psychoanalytic Technique' (1928), describes as the patient's diapason, the capacity to produce or resonate with a pure tone. The diapason expresses Ferenczi's lifelong search for a relational truth, for emotional honesty, openness, and self-disclosure.

Both patient and analyst possess tools of acoustic resonance, a circumstance that helps to explain one of Ferenczi's most highly sophisticated – and most frequently misunderstood – technical propositions: the complementarity of the frustration principle and the relaxation principle. This misunderstanding started with a mistranslation. In his 1928 essay on elasticity, Ferenczi introduced his rule of empathy, bringing with it important modifications to Freud's insistence on frustration, abstinence, and neutrality. When the 1955 English translation of Ferenczi's works referred, however, to the idea of 'indulgence' (Ferenczi, 1929, p. 115) – a translation of his concept of *Nachgiebigkeit* – the significance of empathy began to become lost and Ferenczi's analytic style appeared to be a giving in to the analysand's demands. But as Arnold Rachman has explained, *Nachgiebigkeit* has a strong positive meaning: it does not signify giving in, but rather 'a willingness to give to', a flexibility, suppleness, or pliability (Rachman, 1998, p. 65). In other words, the analyst and patient mutually determine the correct pitch of the therapy.

While it is important to retranslate *Nachgiebigkeit*, it is of even greater importance to recuperate Ferenczi's conception of frustration and relaxation. In his paper on neo-catharsis, the idea of complementarity between the two represents the crux of his notion of the patient's 'economy of suffering' (Ferenczi, 1929, p. 118). He states with striking clarity: 'psychoanalysis employs two opposite methods: it produces heightening of the tension by the frustration it imposes and relaxation by the freedom it allows' (Ferenczi, 1929, p. 115). Ferenczi's 'active technique' is built around the same rhythmic core and presupposes a productive sequencing of tension and relaxation: 'In requiring what is inhibited, and inhibiting what is uninhibited, we hope for a fresh distribution of the patient's psychic, primarily of his libidinal energy that will further the laying bare of the repressed material' (Ferenczi, 1921b, p. 212). From this sequence emerges a new time – a pulsating time that resembles a meandering line. This temporal schema reflects a basic vitality of life. Like the movement of blood to and from the heart, the analyst's 'willingness to give to' alternates with the limitation or prohibition of gratification. A rhythm is thus imprinted on the process; in fact, the analytic process is predicated on the rhythmic capacity of the analytic dyad. Ferenczi therefore introduces a *kairotic* notion of time: both flexibility and restraint must occur at the right time, reacting to the vitalities and the morbidities of the other. Ferenczi's pulsating time is necessarily a time that is responsive to the other: its alternations must be attuned to the patient, composing a 'dialogue of unconsciouses' (Ferenczi, 1932, p. 84).

Ferenczi's pulsating time does not derive from an overpowering, enigmatic, or thin notion of intuition. The genesis of this meandering line can be found in Ferenczi's own biographical and clinical inquiries and in his work with difficult patients (such as Elizabeth Severn, his most well-known case). In his *Clinical Diary*, Ferenczi comments:

> This was the point where I refused to follow him [Freud]. Against his will I began to deal openly with questions of technique. I refused to abuse the patients' trust in this way, and neither did I share his idea that therapy was worthless. I believed rather that therapy was good, but perhaps we were still deficient, and I began to look for our errors. In this search I took several false steps; I went too far with Rank, because on one point (the transference situation) he dazzled me with his new insight. I tried to pursue the Freudian technique of frustration honestly and sincerely to the end (active therapy). Following its failure I tried permissiveness and relaxation, again an exaggeration. In the wake of these two defeats, I am working humanely and naturally, with benevolence, and free from personal prejudices, on the acquisition of knowledge that will allow me to help.
>
> (Ferenczi, 1932, p. 186)

The humane and natural work that Ferenczi refers to here leads to his third concept of time, orchestrated as undulating temporal moves when what is inhibited comes to be required and what is unrestrained becomes inhibited. The meandering line demands a special mental discipline of the analyst; cathexes oscillate between 'identification (analytic object-love) on the one hand and self-control or intellectual activity on the other' (Ferenczi, 1928, p. 98). What results from sustaining this discipline is a chain of kairotic emergence and a model of elasticity: being 'at the right time' (with the other) allows the other to relive the time of trauma and learn to be 'at the right time' with others in turn. The pulsating time of the analytic setting thus breaks into the pulsating time of the patient's life. As Ferenczi states: 'The ideal result of a completed analysis is precisely that elasticity which analytic technique demands of the mental therapist' (Ferenczi, 1928, p. 99).

Achieving this chain of emergence imposes strong exigencies on the analyst. Both frustration and relaxation come with pitfalls and can be abused. The necessity to pursue them in a productive sequence, leading to a better economy of suffering for the patient, only increases these exigencies. In this matter, Ferenczi conducts himself again without many illusions:

> I am of course conscious that this twofold method of frustration and indulgence [*Nachgiebigkeit* in the original] requires from the analyst himself an even greater control than before of counter-transference and counter-resistance. It is no uncommon thing for even those teachers and

> parents who take their task very seriously to be led by imperfectly mastered instincts into excess in either direction. Nothing is easier than to use the principle of frustration in one's relation with patients and children as a cloak for indulgence in one's own unconfessed inclinations. On the other hand, exaggerated forms and quantities of tenderness may subserve one's own, possibly unconscious, libidinal tendencies, rather than the ultimate good of the individual in one's care.
>
> (Ferenczi, 1929, p. 124)

Ferenczi's notions of elasticity and active technique build upon his concept of pulsating time or the meandering line. It is a bold Ferenczian temporality, installing the vitality of life – the dyadic rhythm of frustration and relaxation – at the core of analytic technique.

The drawing below gives a visual representation of the three threads of time discussed above: the tangent-out, the segments and the meandering line.

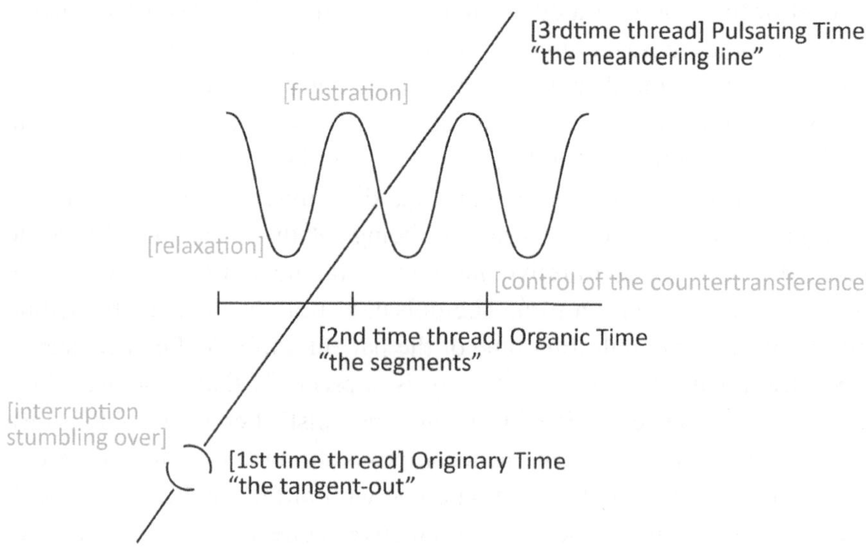

Figure 4.1 Sándor Ferenczi's Times.

Vignette: The Cup of Miriam

A few weeks after the beginning of analysis, Mia announced that she had encountered the 'house of her life'. The building was more than one hundred years old, and it was heavy with traces of a turbulent European twentieth century. At the time of the Second World War, the house belonged to a Jewish woman who was deported and killed in Auschwitz. Mia embarked on a process of reconstructing the history of the house, bringing to the surface the suffering and displacement of her own family during the war as well as raising unanswered questions about her possible hidden Jewish origin. The search to confirm this history became an important occasion for mourning and triggered memories aimed at establishing the authenticity of belonging. Yet, certainty of Jewish origin failed to materialise. The longing to recover her location in history and her family story persisted. Her loss could not be mourned.

In one psychoanalytic session, the story of Mia finding a house intersected with references to the traumatic time of the Holocaust. A significant event took place then. The analyst stood up and gave Mia a Jewish ceremonial cup that had belonged to a member of her own family, some generations ago, and that was placed on a shelf between the couch and the analytic chair. The sequence of gestures – standing up, reaching for the cup, handing the cup, and sharing an element of family history – counted as a sort of stumbling: together, the psychoanalyst and Mia, as individuals and as an analytical pair, we stumbled over a fragment of history. A cup became temporarily (during the time of the session) re-owned, initiating a new cycle of symbolisation. As we see here, it is not only words that slip but also objects: a ritual cup. There is here a movement from the literality of words – 'here is the cup' – to the symbolic load of matter – the cup, actually there, makes a striking invitation beyond itself. Mia held the cup throughout the rest of the session, returning it to the analyst only at the end, when it was put once more in its usual place. During the session, the weight of the need for facts in reconstituting the family story lifted. Despite untraceable details, despite uncertainty, even across the brokenness of a linear story line, loss could be mourned more fully. Not knowing became more bearable. Mia touched an object of the past but, with it, she touched the past as well.[4]

This tactile experience had several reverberations. More than two years after the handing of the cup, Mia associated it to the myth of Miriam, a tangent to an ancestral past. Miriam, the sister of Moses and Aaron, fulfilled a distinctive role in passing on God's word. Moses communicated with God but was unable to speak without stuttering. Aaron, acting as an intermediary between God and the Jewish people, made the words of Moses more clearly discernible. Miriam was a creator: she gave form to the words of Moses in poetry and song. Her voice resonated with natural forces; she could make water spring from dry ground by merely singing and used her gift during the crossing of the desert. According to legend, on the second day of creation a well was made for those who had need of water while journeying through the desert and who were worthy of such a divine gift. Miriam received the well, and after her death, the well was said to have dried up. A contemporary ritual, called *Kos Miryam* (cup of Miriam) by the women who invented it in the early 1970s, centres on the symbolic re-appropriation of a vessel containing waters from Miriam's well. During the ritual, women pass a cup from one to the other, preserving the remembrance of the ancestral well that gave water to those crossing the desert and thus reinvigorating the tradition. As Adelman (1986, 1994) explains, themes that run through Miriam's folklore include those of birth, water, creativity, innovation, risk-taking, and celebration.

What does it mean to pass on a container? It is a risky and paradoxical gesture that disturbs the dichotomy active/passive and confers a sense of mutuality on the analytic setting and analytic relationship. To hand over a container means that the container, apart from performing its 'holding' role, will itself need to be held or supported in all its enigmatic weight. The ritual cup becomes central to a cycle of symbolisation: it is given; it is held; it is retrieved. It functions as a material metaphor, as a 'third space' (Benjamin, 1988) between the analyst and the analysand.

Polyphonies of time run through the handing of the cup. A strong tangent was drawn when the analysand associated the episode with the myth of Miriam. Ancestral time is not only pre-catastrophic, as Ferenczi might argue, but it encompasses concentric containments: a cup, within a cup, within another cup. This concentricity invites a new psychoanalytic language, one that allows us to envisage intergenerational transmissions and, even more particularly, generosities between women. As Adrienne Rich wrote in *Of Woman Born*, 'Until a strong line of love, confirmation, and example stretches from mother to daughter, from woman to woman across the generations, women will still be wandering in the wilderness' (Rich, 1976, p. 246). The myth of Jocasta has perhaps exhausted its creativities as a reference in psychoanalysis for construing women and femininity; the encounter with Miriam, therefore, is refreshing. It seems we are in the presence of a feminine Orpheus – who makes nature resonate, who accomplishes her work by the powers of her voice, who creates poetry and song, and who is endowed with both a passive and active generativity. If Jocasta is the invitation to not questioning and not knowing, Miriam stands for the continual reinvention of tradition. She does not turn against her legacies but uses them for creating new form.

The second time thread I discussed above – the segmented, phased conception of transference and countertransference – was also present with the cup. As this event occurred towards the beginning of the analysis, the analyst's identification with the patient's pain was especially strong. Elements of a shared history were allowed to function as grounds for a therapeutic alliance.

Finally, the third thread of time pulsated within this scene as well. The passive/active act of giving a container intervened in a heightened moment of tension when several threads of traumatic time were condensed in Mia's discourse. By taking a risk and giving Mia the ceremonial cup, the analyst lowered the tension, orchestrating a moment of relaxation that enabled a differentiation of the threads of traumatic time. Mia acknowledged more of her psychic pain and discerned more traces of historical trauma. To touch those times in one moment was a political act in its widest sense. With it, there appeared a fragment of all times that ever were and a flickering trace of innumerable times to come.

On the Position of the Analyst

Having embarked on this journey through various threads of time, we can argue that one of the most important – if not the most important – functions of the analyst is to re-establish the polyphony of time, or the 'polyphony of polyphonies' (Deleuze, 1988). In the previous chapter, while looking at the Orpha fragment of the psyche and its times, we discerned its associations with an eternal present and with the impossibility of the complex temporality of the *Nachträglichkeit*. With Orpha, time is just a single flat surface which contains all the actors, acts, and scenes. The analyst's intervention is that of inhabiting, with the patient, a polyphonic temporality, one where there is present, but also deep past, and recent past, and conditional future, and distant future, and many other times that are yet to be named. Among all these times, the pre-traumatic time is a privileged one. Accessing it is not akin to establishing the truth and authenticity of the trauma scene:

instead, pre-traumatic time is itself a construction, a potential time, one that emerges at the intersection of what could have been and what might yet be. As Ferenczi (1932, p. 27) notes: 'The end result of the analysis of transference and countertransference may be the establishment of a kind, dispassionate atmosphere, such as may well have existed in pre-traumatic times'. Through the analysis of transference and of countertransference, the analytic position becomes coded as that which reignites time as polyphony.

A second important clue in relation to the position of the analyst is that it defines itself in relation to the fragment, rather than to the whole. Having discussed many facets of psychic splitting and fragmentation, we can argue that the analyst works with and from a consciousness of fragments that becomes a practice and a craft. Analysis is work with and across fragments of experience. The analyst, in the best of scenarios, has traversed some of the illusions of wholeness that animate us, including Orphic hallucinations of wholeness and transcendence. Some interpretations – that in my experience patients can make extraordinarily good use of – point precisely to the ego's being in fragments but also to how some of the voices of the fragments can be discerned and worked with. Other interpretations engage the patient's longing for wholeness and yet do not let her linger in a state of hallucinating pre-traumatic tenderness. The analyst can acknowledge both that the patient is in fragments and that they are longing for wholeness and recovery of the 'lost' parts of the ego. Furthermore, the analyst acknowledges her own state of psychic fragmentation. As Ferenczi (1932, p. 13) insightfully writes in the *Clinical Diary*, 'Our psyche [as analysts], too, is more or less fragmented and in pieces, [...] especially after expending so much libido'.

A third clue in relation to the position of the analyst refers to the centrality of analogy. We can say that the analysis is a place for the intensification of analogy. The work with analogies (or comparison between comparisons, or double comparisons, which establish relations between relations) is so important because the unconscious operates by analogies – alongside dreams, mistakes and symptomatic acts. The grammatical operator 'is like' thus has a key role in the unconscious. The formula 'what A is to B, Y is to Z' is another way of expressing this. Analogy and its analysis also contribute to re-establishing the polyphony of times. Not all sets of elements (A, B, Y, and Z) belong to the same time horizon. Analogy is by definition a psychic process that references multiple times. The analyst has a few special entry points to the intensifying of analogies, as she can refer to what the patient said or did in a multiplicity of previous analytic sessions. The result is a kind of weaving across sessions with multiple time knots and with links across time that were not possible before. We can imagine the analyst's grammar here as: 'What you are saying now *is like* what you said two months ago' or 'This episode *is like* the story you told me three weeks ago'.

After having organised Ferenczi's insights on the analyst's times into three different temporal threads – originary time, organic time and pulsating time – it is meaningful to go on a condensed journey into his main contributions to psychoanalytic technique. In so doing, we can arrive at some further insights about the position of the analyst. Ferenczi has produced a core body of work on issues of technique in which we can also trace the development of his unique vocabulary: it goes from tact, sincerity, hypocrisy, and horizontality to active psychoanalytic technique, the elasticity of technique, the principle of relaxation and neo-catharsis, mutuality and mutual analysis, and the role of regression and reliving in the psychoanalytic process. The key writings to consider here are: the early 1919 text 'On the technique of psycho-analysis'; the texts that debate each other on 'active technique'; 'The further development of active therapy in psychoanalysis' of 1920 and 'Contra-indications to the "active" psychoanalytic technique' of 1921; the notable 1925 monograph co-authored with Otto Rank, *The Development of Psycho-Analytic Technique*; the extraordinary and more mature pair of texts from 1928, 'The elasticity of psychoanalytic technique' and 'The principle of relaxation and neo-catharsis', 1929; and of course, the *Clinical Diary*, written in 1932, containing rich insights into hypocrisy, mutuality and regression.[5]

Within the *Clinical Diary* itself, I would point the reader to a selection of entries that are crucial in reconstituting the genealogy of the mutual analysis experiment as well as in grasping the theoretical construction of 'mutuality' itself. These are the entries of 17 January 1932, 'Mutual analysis and the limits of its application'; 6 March 1932, 'Mutuality'; 5 May 1932, 'Case of R.N.'; 12 May 1932, 'Technique: error (emotion instead of objectivity): (1) commit, (2) confess, (3) correct'; and 18 June 1932, 'A new stage in mutuality'. In the previous chapter, I showed how patient Elizabeth Severn is a key presence in the formulation of these ideas on mutuality to the extent that Ferenczi's trauma theory and theory of countertransference can be considered a co-construction (see Rachman, 2017).

Ferenczi is rightly considered a precursor of the contemporary commitment to working on the countertransference of the analyst to the patient. The 'discovery of countertransference' can be traced back to an exchange between Freud and Jung. The word appears for the first time in an exchange of letters between the two about Jung's feelings and acting out in relation to Sabina Spielrein; shortly after this, it becomes part of psychoanalytic language. André Haynal (1999) has aptly followed the concept 'travelling' through various psychoanalytic traditions. As far as the Budapest School of Psychoanalysis is concerned, countertransference was given a privileged place very early on, in the 1920s, and it was the focus of the clinical seminar led by Vilma Kovács. The intense search for ways of working on the countertransference is reflected in the Budapest model of supervision. In this model, out of the two training cases that any analyst must receive supervision for, the first training case was supervised by one's own analyst while the second training case was supervised by a different analyst. As I have shown elsewhere (Soreanu, 2019), far from marking a lack of reflexivity on the dangers that this practice bears in relation to transforming the candidate's analyst into a figure of hyper-authority, this model was developed as a good-enough solution to the problem of placing countertransference at the centre of the psychoanalytic dispositif and at the centre of the transmission of psychoanalytic knowledge.

Ferenczi's *Clinical Diary* paints the picture of a 'system' made up by transference and countertransference considered together, or of a 'structure' erected by two parties, in which the analyst's contribution is the counterpart of the analysand's (Haynal, 1999). The analyst thus becomes one of the principal subjects; his countertransference is no longer 'counter' in the sense of being 'against' but is 'with' the patient. Countertransference can even be seen as *preceding* the transference, as I argued above. Furthermore, Ferenczi is notoriously the first to have stressed the importance of the analysis of the analyst. It is only through a deep personal analysis that the psychoanalyst can diminish or adequately address the obstacles to the treatment that originate in his own psychic functioning and traumatic marks or narcissistic marks. Many different lines from the *Clinical Diary* can support this account: 'Analysts should be analysed *better, not* worse, than patients'; 'Mutual analysis: only a last resort! Proper analysis by a stranger, without any obligation, would be better'; and 'The best analyst is the patient who has been cured' (Ferenczi, 1932, p. 115).

Another early intervention into the technical knowledge in psychoanalysis comes in the form of an anticipation of the famous Kleinian 'here-and-now' technique. In the 1924 monograph co-authored by Ferenczi and Rank (1925), *The Development of Psycho-Analytic Technique*, they argue that the point of analysis is not to prove the 'correctness of theory'. Rather, it 'consists in understanding and interpreting every expression of the patient above all as a reaction to the present analytical situation (defence against, or recognition of the expositions of the analyst, emotional reactions to these, etc)'. This early version of 'here-and-now' interpretation was supposed to address not only the actions of the patient in the consulting room but also the use the patient makes, or fails to make, of the analyst's thinking. The patient can either defend against the analyst's mind, insights and presence; or they can recognise and make use of the analysts thinking process while accepting it as different from their own. These ideas are similar to Betty Joseph's (2013) work that came much later on.

For Ferenczi, sensitivity – or tact – is a fundamental *instrument* of the analytic process and of the analyst's participation in it – her organ of perception. This sensitivity must be maintained and cared for – in contrast to an analytic attitude of 'desperately rigid clinging to a theoretical approach' (Ferenczi, 1932, p. 1). It is through this sensitivity that the analyst can strive to maintain the horizontality of the analytic situation while holding hierarchical impulses in check. Tact also comes into play when it comes to unavoidable errors made by the analyst. Making errors as such is not damaging to the analytic process: on the contrary, an error opens up the space for a scene of recognition. When the error is not denied, or put 'into' the patient, it can strengthen the analysis:

> One could almost say that the more weaknesses an analyst has, which lead to greater or lesser mistakes and errors but which are then uncovered and treated in the course of [...] analysis, the more likely the analysis is to rest on profound and realistic foundations.
>
> (Ferenczi, 1932, p. 15)

However, the analyst's superego often gets in the way of this productive way of balancing the analysis through the errors of the analyst. The analyst's superego can produce various distortions: it can make it difficult to admit to any errors; or, due to a powerful sense of guilt, it can lead to demonstrations of 'superkindness' which overcompensate for any negative feelings that the analyst might experience in relation to the patient. In his text on 'The elasticity of psychoanalytic technique', Ferenczi tells us: 'One must never be ashamed unreservedly to confess one's own mistakes. It must never be forgotten that analysis is no suggestive process, primarily dependent on the physician's reputation and infallibility. All that it calls for is confidence in the physician's frankness and honesty, which does not suffer from the frank confession of mistakes' (Ferenczi, 1928, p. 95).

One of the most unusual characteristics of the *Clinical Diary* – and of other earlier writings on technique – is Ferenczi's ability to acknowledge and discuss his own mistakes or failed technical experimentations. This remains a rare quality in clinical writing even in our own times. His 1919, 1920 and 1921 papers touching on 'active technique' are on a trajectory in which Ferenczi first experiments with elements of active technique – where he occasionally introduces forms of 'instruction' in relation to some of the symptoms of his patients – only to afterwards conclude that active technique has considerable counterindications, and interpretation remains the better path. By 'active technique', I don't refer here to giving patients concrete advice or making direct suggestions. Instead, Freud's choice of setting a date for the finishing of his analysis with Wolf Man is a very good instance of working with active technique. The setting of an end date 'acts' on the analysis, perhaps accelerating something in the treatment. As mentioned, Ferenczi recognised the serious limitations of introducing elements of active technique in the analytic process:

> I wish therefore so far as possible to repeat, and this time in unmistakable fashion, that 'activity' unquestionably stimulates the resistance of the patient in so far as it seeks to increase the psychical tension by painful frustrations, injunctions, and prohibitions, and so gain new material. That is to say, the ego of the patient runs counter to the analyst.
>
> (Ferenczi, 1921b, p. 218)

If the active mandates are bound to stimulate resistance, what remains as the main instrument of the analyst is a kind of modulating presence, a pliability of the libido, a capacity to step forward or step back, in tune with the analysand.

It is this image of pliability and the capacity of being with that is the centre of another of Ferenczi's (1928) key ideas on technique: the 'elasticity of technique'. Ferenczi is inspired by one of his patients' observations when thinking through the analyst's pliability:

> A patient of mine once spoke of the 'elasticity of analytic technique', a phrase which I fully accept. The analyst, like an elastic band, must yield to the patient's pull, but without ceasing to pull in his own direction, so long as one position or the other has not been conclusively demonstrated to be untenable.
>
> (Ferenczi, 1928, p. 95)

It is the mobility of the analyst's libido, acquired in the course of their own personal analysis, that produces this effect of elasticity or of a particular combination of force and counterforce that is productive for the psychoanalytic process.

As I pointed out in a previous chapter, both Ferenczi and Michael Balint have a strong interest in the possibility of a 'benign regression' (Bálint, 1968) in the psychoanalytic process, where the patient can get in touch with traumatic marks and even parts of the psyche which have become radically separated from the conscious ego. What enables these difficult regressive states to become part of an analytic construction between the patient and the analyst is precisely the analyst's different *position* in relation to the scene of trauma: one that acknowledges the magnitude of suffering and brings recognition. In the presence of the analyst, sometime in the form of trance-like states, the patient gets in touch with 'physical memory symbols' (Ferenczi, 1929, p. 119) – currents of affect inscribed in the body, its parts and its organs, affective traces and poignant residues of the trauma scene – which have not yet been linked up to verbal signifiers or have not been fantasised into. When such odd marks, residues, and sections of scenes animated by affect get relived in the consulting room, a kind of *reconstruction* of the past takes place, and this reconstructed past has a stronger feeling of reality and concreteness to it than the patient ever experienced before. The result *feels* like a memory, although it is not an exact account of the trauma scene.

This kind of regression will make possible a 'new beginning' – a term that Michael Bálint (1968) will later put at the centre of his propositions on 'benign regression' and 'the basic fault'. Ferenczi (1929) calls this regression 'neo-catharsis'. What is repeated in this state of regression is the original conflict between the ego and the environment, and the painful intrapsychic solutions found for this conflict, in search of a fresh resolution. The analyst is positioned as a part of this 'new beginning'; in fact, the psychic reconstruction that it entails can only be attained if the analyst practices a particular sort of *clinical sincerity* which is in direct contrast to the denial that the patient would have experienced in childhood. This clinical sincerity (the counterpoint of *professional hypocrisy*) makes it possible for the patient to experience the traumatic events of the past as thoughts or as objective memories, not only as hallucinatory reproductions. The new position of clinical sincerity taken by the analyst is akin to a new environment, or a set of 'new conditions', which can lead to a new psychic resolution for the patient and a new re-arrangement of the psychic fragments. Ferenczi argues that

> [t]he most essential aspect of the altered repetition is the relinquishing of one own's rigid authority and the hostility hidden in it. The relief that is obtained thereby is then not transient and the convictions derived in this way are also more deeply rooted.
>
> (Ferenczi, 1932, p. 108)

In other words, the analyst will experiment with not taking a position of authority that demands submission. This position is *different* from the situation in childhood, which was one of suggestion and the emergence of infantile obedience, in the form of a psychic scene played and replayed between a small vulnerable being and a big overpowering one. In the *Clinical Diary*, Ferenczi refers to mutuality as an 'antidote' to the hypnotic lies of childhood. His register of terms in describing the analyst's intervention includes ideas such as *demechanisation* or *dehypnotising*, implying a (partial) reversibility of psychic processes of fragmentation. The psychic state of functioning as an 'automaton' – which was produced in the process of identifying with the aggressor – is at least in part reversible given the experience of sensitive listening and recognition of suffering in the analytic frame. What Ferenczi suggests is that in the analysis the scene of trauma is re-staged in new psychic circumstances:

> the recognition and assertion of one own's self as a genuinely existing, a valuable entity of a given size, shape, and significance – is attainable only when the positive interest of the environment, let us say libido,

> guarantees the stability of that form of personality by means of external pressure, so to speak. Without such a counter-pressure, let us say counterlove [*Gegenliebe*], the individual tends to explode, to dissolve itself in the universe, perhaps to die.
>
> (Ferenczi, 1932, p. 129)

*

It often seems to me that I have spent the last 12 years, while seated in the analytic chair, in a state of counter-love. Ferenczi was my day-to-day companion across space and time. I drew his consulting room close to my own as if we had been sharing a waiting room. He helped me to fine-tune any instrument I ever had or tried out, perhaps as one tunes a chord instrument. He even helped me in naming and describing this singular affect: *counter-love*. Counter-love is for me associated with a state of resistance to the identification with the aggressor. Counter-love also brings a psychic temporality I call *conditional future perfect*. No language I speak contains conditional future perfect among the times of the verb: it is a necessary invention. It refers to a psychic action undertaken *in the name of a time when the Other would have done less harm*. It is a humble time, a time of self-limitation, a time of no illusions, no full 'reparation' or 'integration'. It is a time of partial reconstruction, working with whatever exists 'on the table' of the analysis. To inhabit the world in the conditional future perfect is to ask: what if there is a way to do less harm? What would less harm have looked like then? And what might it look like now?

Notes

1 Green wrote: 'Modern psychoanalysis has turned away from the search for the multiple paths necessary for temporal construction, perhaps owing to deceptions resulting from the speculative exercise which endeavoured to answer enigmas. To replace it, it only found, in my view, impoverishing solutions, such as the technique "here and now", which comprised no fewer hazardous speculations by relating everything to a present arising from the thought of the analyst alone, no less debatable in the forms that it was supposed to take' (2009, p. 16).

2 Freud wrote to Ferenczi on 3 December 1910: 'I see destiny approaching inexorably, and I note that it has designated you to bring to light mysticism and the like, and that it would be just as futile as it is hard-hearted to keep you from it. Still, I think we ought to venture to slow it down. I would like to request that you continue to research in secrecy for two full years and don't come out until 1913; then, certainly, in the Jahrbuch, openly and aboveboard. You know my practical reasons against it and my secret painful sensitivities' (in Freud et al., 1993, pp. 239–240).

3 It would be worthwhile to examine the resonances between Ferenczi's analogical epistemology and Gregory Bateson's epistemology of metaphor (see Bateson & Bateson,

1987). For Bateson, metaphor involves the operations of homology, empathy, and abduction, allowing one to gain access to the pattern that connects different strata of reality.

4 In *Á la recherche du temps perdu*, Marcel Proust revised Bergson's notion of selective memory by introducing involuntary memory, which is encountered through contingency. Stumbling over the smell of a madeleine cake, a memory of growing up in Combray comes to the fore. For Walter Benjamin (1973), involuntary memory is not willed but is encountered through a shock or surprise.

5 See Ferenczi (1919, 1920, 1921b, 1928, 1929, 1932) and Ferenczi and Rank (1925).

References

Adelman, P. V. (1986). *Miriam's Well: Rituals for Jewish Women around the Year.* New York, NY: Bilbio Press.

Adelman, P. V. (1994). A drink from Miriam's cup: Invention of tradition among Jewish women. *Journal of Feminist Studies in Religion*, 10(2): 151–166.

Arlow, J. A. (1984). Disturbances of the sense of time, with special reference to the experience of timelessness. *Psychoanalytic Quarterly*, 53: 13–37.

Arlow, J. A. (1986). Psychoanalysis and time. *Journal of the American Psychoanalytic Association*, 34: 507–528.

Bálint, M. (1968). *The Basic Fault. Therapeutic Aspects of Regression.* London: Tavistock.

Bateson, G., & Bateson, M. C. (1987). *Angels Fear: Toward an Epistemology of the Sacred.* New York, NY: Macmillan.

Benjamin, J. (1988). *The Bonds of Love.* New York, NY: Pantheon.

Benjamin, W. (1973). *Charles Baudelaire: A Lyric Poet in the Era of High Capitalism* (transl. by H. Zohn). London: New Left Books.

Bion, W. R. (1970). *Attention and Interpretation: A Scientific Approach to Insight in Psychoanalysis and Groups.* London: Tavistock.

Birksted-Breen, D. (2012). Taking time: The tempo of psychoanalysis. *International Journal of Psychoanalysis*, 93: 819–35.

Botella, C., & Botella, S. (2005). *The Work of Psychic Figurability: Mental States Without Representation* (transl. by A. Weller, with M. Zerbib). London: Routledge.

Cabré, l. J. M. (2008). The psychoanalytic conception of trauma in Ferenczi and the question of temporality. *American Journal of Psychoanalysis*, 68: 43–49.

Deleuze, G. (1985). *Spinoza et le problème de l expression.* Paris: PUF.

Deleuze, G. (1988). *Le Pli: Leibniz et la Baroque*. Paris: Minuit.

Ferenczi, S. (1899). Spiritism. *Psychoanalytic Review*, 50A: 139–144, 1963.

Ferenczi, S. (1913). The ontogenesis of symbols. In: *Final Contributions to the Problems and Methods of Psycho-analysis* (transl. by E. Mosbacher, pp. 276–281 London: Karnac, 1994.

Ferenczi, S. (1919). On the technique of psychoanalysis. In: *Further Contributions to the Theory and Technique of Psycho-analysis* (transl. by J. I. Suttie, pp. 89–104). London: Karnac, 1994.

Ferenczi, S. (1920). The further development of an active therapy in psycho-analysis. In: *Further Contributions to the Theory and Technique of Psycho-analysis* (transl. by J. I. Suttie, pp. 198–217). London: Karnac, 1994.

Ferenczi, S. (1921a). The symbolism of the bridge. In: *Further Contributions to the Theory and Technique of Psycho-analysis* (transl. by J. I. Suttie, pp. 352–356). London: Karnac, 1994.
Ferenczi, S. (1921b). Contra-indications to the 'active' psychoanalytic technique. In: *Further Contributions to the Theory and Technique of Psycho-analysis* (transl. by J. I. Suttie, pp. 218–230). London: Karnac, 1994.
Ferenczi, S. (1924). *Thalassa. A Theory of Genitality* (transl. by H. A. Bunker). London & New York, NY: Karnac, 1989.
Ferenczi, S. (1928). The elasticity of psycho-analytic technique. In: *Final contributions to the Problems and Methods of Psycho-analysis* (transl. by E. Mosbacher, pp. 87–101). London: Karnac, 1994.
Ferenczi, S. (1929). The principle of relaxation and neocatharsis. In: *Final Contributions to the Problems and Methods of Psycho-analysis* (transl. by E. Mosbacher, pp. 108–125). London: Karnac, 1994.
Ferenczi, S. (1932). *The Clinical Diary of Sándor Ferenczi*, ed. by J. Dupont (transl. by M. Bálint & N. Z. Jackson). Cambridge, MA: Harvard University Press, 1995.
Ferenczi, S., & Rank, O. (1925). *The Development of Psychoanalysis* (transl. by C. Newton). New York, NY: Nervous and Mental Disease Publishing Company.
Freud, S. (1937). Constructions in analysis. In: *Standard Edition* (Vol. 23, pp. 255–269). London: Hogarth Press.
Freud, S., Ferenczi, S., Brabant, E., Falzeder, E., & Haynal, A. (eds) (1993). *The Correspondence of Sigmund Freud and Sándor Ferenczi, Vol. 1, 1908–1914* (transl. by P. T. Hoffer). Cambridge, MA: Belknap Press/Harvard University Press.
Frosh, S. (2012). Hauntings: Psychoanalysis and ghostly transmission. *American Imago*, 69: 241–264.
Green, A. (2000). *Le Temps éclaté.* Paris: Éditions de Minuit.
Green, A. (2009). From the ignorance of time to the murder of time: From the murder of time to the misrecognition of temporality in psychoanalysis (transl. by A. Weller). In: I. Glocer Fiorini & J. Canestri (eds), *The Experience of Time: Psychoanalytic Perspectives* (pp. 1–20). London: Karnac.
Guattari, F. (2011). *The Machinic Unconscious: Essays in Schizoanalysis* (transl. by T. Adkins). Los Angeles, CA: Semiotext(e).
Gyimesi, J. (2012). Sándor Ferenczi and the problem of telepathy. *History of the Human Sciences*, 25(2): 131–148.
Hartocollis, P. (1972). Time as a dimension of affects. *Journal of the American Psychoanalytic Association*, 20: 92–108.
Hartocollis, P. (1974). Origins of time: A reconstruction of ontogenetic development of the sense of time based on object-relations theory. *The Psychoanalytic Quarterly*, 43: 243–261.
Hartocollis, P. (1983). *Time and Timelessness: The Varieties of Temporal Experience.* New York, NY: International Universities Press.
Hartocollis, P. (2003). Time and the psychoanalytic situation. *The Psychoanalytic Quarterly*, 72: 939–957.
Haynal, A. (1999). The countertransference in the work of Ferenczi. *American Journal of Psychoanalysis*, 59(4): 315–331.
Joseph, B. (2013). Here and now: My perspective. *International Journal of Psychoanalysis*, 94(1): 1–5.

Lacan, J. (1988). Logical time and the assertion of anticipated certainty: A new sophism (transl. by B. Fink & M. Silver). *Newsletter of the Freudian Field*, 2(2): 4–22.
Laget, A. (1995). *Freud et le temps.* Lyon: Presses universitaires de Lyon.
Ogden, T. H. (1997). Reverie and metaphor: Some thoughts on how I work as a psychoanalyst. *International Journal of Psychoanalysis*, 78: 719–732.
Pelbart, P. P. (2010). *O tempo não-reconciliado.* São Paulo: Perspectiva.
Perelberg, R. J. (2008). *Time, Space and Phantasy.* London: Routledge.
Rachman, A. (1998). Ferenczi's relaxation principle and the issue of therapeutic responsiveness. *American Journal of Psychoanalysis*, 58: 63–81.
Rachman, A. (2017). *Elizabeth Severn: The 'Evil Genius' of Psychoanalysis*. London: Routledge.
Rich, A. C. (1976). *Of Woman Born: Motherhood as Experience and Institution.* New York, NY: W.W. Norton & Company.□□□□□□□□
Rickman, J. (1933). Obituary: Sándor Ferenczi. *Proceedings of the Society for Psychical Research*, 33: 124–125.
Sabbadini, A. (1989). Boundaries of timelessness: Some thoughts about the temporal dimension of psychoanalytic space. *International Journal of Psychoanalysis*, 70: 305–313.
Sabbadini, A. (2014). *Boundaries and Bridges: Perspectives on Time and Space in Psychoanalysis.* London: Karnac.
Soreanu, R. (2019). Supervision for our times: Countertransference and the rich legacy of the Budapest School. *The American Journal of Psychoanalysis*, 79(3): 329–351.
Winnicott, D. W. (1971). *Playing and Reality.* London: Tavistock.

Coda

A Few Explosions

> Our Lady of the Couch, pray for us.
> Our Lady of the Symptom, pray for us.
> Our Lady of the Unconscious, pray for us.
> Our Lady of Choice of Object, pray for us.
> Our Lady of the Mirror Phase, pray for us.
> Our Lady of the Death Drive, pray for us.
> Our Lady of the Libido, pray for us.
>
> (Paul B. Preciado, *Dysphoria Mundi*, 2025, p. 129)

In the last few months, I kept returning to the 'Funeral Prayer', written by Paul B. Preciado in his recent book *Dysphoria Mundi.* I reproduce part of it above, but invite the reader to encounter it in full: it references many more psychoanalytic objects, terms and anchors alongside 'Our Lady of the Couch'. Why do philosophers need to pray for psychoanalysis? This ironic funeral prayer is addressed, I believe, to an institutional and ritualised psychoanalysis, invested in preserving rigid norms and thus actively harming non-normative lives and experiences. This psychoanalysis is frozen and deadening. These days, I wonder in which way we can reconstruct psychoanalytic objects, theories and practices, in the name of an *infrastructural psychoanalysis* (Soreanu & Minozzo, 2024; Berlant, 2022), one that looks at institutions 'slantwise', is inclined to work with multiple transferences, can traverse ambivalences, and has a consistent orientation to marginal lives, to outcast objects, to detritus and scraps. In these pages, I regarded reusing and repurposing as core psychic acts, which turn psychoanalysis into a kind of gleaning, and also into a necessarily *minor* psychoanalysis. This minor psychoanalysis can be part of a radical political ecology that places the question of the living and desiring body at its centre.

DOI: 10.4324/9781032715926-6

Paul B. Preciado (2025, p. 47) writes about the current global time of crisis: 'the new universality consists in feeling that the living body, our body, is exploding'. Many of my patients talk about different kinds of explosions, pulverisations, atomisations, states of being suspended, up in the air. Remember my patient Ava, who asked me: 'Do you know that painting by Dali? It's a Renaissance girl-head exploding? That's how I feel, most of the time, in pieces and like all my organs are out of place…'. Faced with so many psychic and somatic explosions, and in the frame of actual explosions, in Gaza, Ukraine, Sudan or Myanmar, what can psychoanalysts do?

In these pages, the answer I gave is: consider the radical plasticity of the psyche and its many surprising fractures, splits, leakages, but also new formations, protective membranes, expansions, contagions, and inner growths. In Greek, *plastikos* refers to the capacity to be shaped or moulded, and it is derived from *plastos*, which means malleable or open to transformation. In her book *Plasticity: The Promise of Explosion*, Catherine Malabou (2022) comments on Freud's inability (in 'Beyond the Pleasure Principle') to conceive of negative plasticity, or destructive plasticity, or of an event of annihilation that is also an event of forming. In turning to Ferenczi, I aimed not only to be curious about negative plasticity, but to further qualify moments of fragmentation when life is present in death, and death is present in life. Strange processes and formations such as Orpha, teratoma, autotomy and teleplasty point to an annihilation that is bound up with surviving and with creating something new. I have found that pondering radical plasticity is the best companion to the psychoanalytic consulting room of our times, and it helps in being-with patients who feel that their living body is exploding.

Ferenczi is a good 'accomplice' in the task of considering radical plasticity because he is a complexity theorist, in the sense of allowing us to imagine a stratified ontology where different strata of reality (and of the psyche) are characterised by different unique logics, and they lean on one another, without ever being reducible to one another. This is why I have spoken of the different 'registers' of the unconscious and of memory. Ferenczi is a good 'accomplice' also because he resonates and can fruitfully be read alongside psychoanalysts and philosophers that make up an archipelago of affinities in facing the forms of suffering of our times. I am thinking here of Cornelius Castoriadis (on the radical imagination and the creation of new drives), André Green (on the function of the negative), René Roussillon (on splitting and the non-symbolic), Julia Kristeva (on the semiotic and the chora), Jean Laplanche (on the fundamental anthropological situation and asymmetry), Frantz Fanon (on fragmentation) and Jacques Lacan (on *le corps morcelé*). I am also thinking of Spinoza (on the body), Walter Benjamin (on mimetism and language), Gilles Deleuze and Félix Guattari (on the plurality of semiotic codes), Gregory Bateson (on the adjustive ability of the soma), José Gil (on the fluctuating signifier and the language of the body), Michel Serres (on interruption and the event), Catherine Malabou (on plasticity), Édouard Glissant (on shared knowledge), Karen Barad (on diffractive readings) and Donna Haraway (on tentacular knowledge and so much more). Within this archipelago, many more compositions are possible around questions such as: What can a fragment do? What can a turbulence create or enable? What does it mean to relate ethically to the Other within a paradigm of asymmetric relationality – while knowing that the scene of an encounter between large and small, between rigid and plastic, between overpowering and fragile is something that keeps returning?

Ferenczi is a good 'accomplice' in the clinic of our times because he is overwhelmingly concerned with difference and singularity. While his metapsychological constructs are strong and necessary, and while by starting from his insights we can articulate a metapsychology of fragmented psyches, it seems that for him the state of fragmentation of each patient mobilises a singular theoretical-clinical response, or arrangement, or even a dedicated language. Let us turn to the way he captures the fragmented psyche of his patient Elizabeth Severn in the *Clinical Diary*, bringing a montage made of a conscious part of the ego, radically severed from the rest of the psyche; a de-libidinised part of the ego that was pushed back into the id; a part of the id bearing traumatic marks that can appear in traumatic dreams and states of regression in the analysis; and a 'deep id', which remains resistant to symbolisation. In his own words:

> She managed, however, as if by a miracle, to get this being back on its feet, shattered as it was to its very atoms, and thus procured a sort of artificial psyche for this body forcibly brought back to life. From now on the 'individuum', superficially regarded, consists of the following parts: (a) uppermost, a capable, active human being with a precisely – perhaps a little too precisely – regulated mechanism; (b) behind this, a being that does not wish to have anything more to do with life; (c) behind this murdered ego, the ashes of earlier mental sufferings, which

> are rekindled every night by the fire of suffering; (d) this suffering itself as a separate mass of affect, without content and unconscious, the remains of the actual person.
>
> (Ferenczi, 1932, p. 10)

There is one more type of explosion that I would like to consider. It is the necessary explosion of the psychoanalytic author. Indeed, I believe there is no author when it comes to psychoanalytic writing. There is perhaps only an approximation, a rendition, a searching. Psychoanalytic *insight* involves the more-than-one and different types of work done beyond the analyst: dream-work by the patient, attempts at working-through, the work of the dyad in transference/countertransference. *Writing* all this up would need to involve the more-than-one as well, but there are not many ways to achieve this, ethically or in practice. I have tried to transcribe, translate and transubstantiate, in relative solitude, what was passed over to me by Others. I have also tried to swerve away from the illusion that the analyst is a coherent and integrated subject. Ferenczi understood this sort of explosion: 'Our psyche [as analysts], too, is more or less fragmented and in pieces, [...] especially after expending so much libido [...]' (Ferenczi, 1932, p. 13).

A collage by Dada artist Hannah Höch, who has been my companion in rereading Ferenczi, comes to mind. It is her work 'Der Strauß', which she started in 1929 and completed in 1965.[1] In this collage, Höch presents the viewer with a vibrantly coloured bouquet made out of eyes, in a montage that is both playfully extravagant and uncanny. What to do with a bunch of eyes, looking somewhat like an explosion of an individual eye? A radical operation needs to be performed on the White Man's individual gaze: to explode it, to split it up, to undo it via forms of diffraction. We might need to find our way to the root of the French word for 'gaze', *regard*, which originally did not refer strictly to the act of seeing, but to watchfulness, watching over, expectation, concern, and even keeping safe. This line of associations is strengthened by the prefix re-, suggesting a recurrent watchfulness, a redoubling of the act, a return to concern.

In the root of this word, like in Hannah Höch's collage, there is a reference to something more-than-seeing, in excess of seeing, which can undo a cold and mortifying gaze. Jakob Staberg (2023) writes about the 'tactile eye' of the psychoanalyst and about a mode of haptic visuality. I wrote of Ferenczi as a 'tentacular' psychoanalyst and thinker: feeling, trying, experimenting, hesitating, advancing, retracting, revising; always relying on more than one sense or to a point of intersection between the senses, a synaesthesia. Kwame Yonatan Poli dos Santos (2023) speaks of 'listening with the gaze' [*escutar com o olhar*], a particular type of listening that the psychoanalyst relies on, so as to be able to hear the suffering of the patient, including the suffering that is the consequence of living in the 'colonial matrix'. He suggests that the analyst needs to invent new organs for listening – organs beyond sensorial activity – in order to follow the complicated mixings and transpositions of psychic registers that happen in the psychoanalytic frame and while living in a racialised society. What might we be able to see with a tactile eye?

In asking this, I remember that my patient Ava told me once that as a child living in a poor neighbourhood and while playing on the streets, she found in the rubbish a copy of Freud's *Interpretation of Dreams.* This scrap object, discarded and re-found, was part of the way she later on found her way to my consulting room – in the social clinic where I was seeing patients at that time – and to her capacity to dream. An unlikely event led to a creative composition. In a time of explosions, what we are left with is the inclination to go through the detritus, in the hope of finding something usable.

Note

1 The work is available at: https://www.artchive.com/artwork/strauss-hannah-hoch-1965/. Accessed 25 July 2025.

References

Berlant, L. (2022). *On the Inconvenience of Other People*. Durham, NC: Duke University Press.

Ferenczi, S. (1932). *The Clinical Diary of Sándor Ferenczi*, ed. by J. Dupont (transl. by M. Bálint & N. Z. Jackson). Cambridge, MA: Harvard University Press, 1995.

Malabou, C. (2022). *Plasticity: The Promise of Explosion*. Edinburgh: Edinburgh University Press.

Poli dos Santos, K. Y. (2023). *Por um Fio: Uma Escuta das Diásporas Pulsionais.* Curitiba: Editora Calligraphie.

Preciado, P. B. (2025). *Dysphoria Mundi.* London: Fitzcarraldo Editions.

Soreanu, R., & Minozzo, A. (2024). Manifesto for infrastructural thinking: Living with psychoanalysis in a glitch. *Psychoanalysis, Culture & Society*, 29(3): 323–342.

Staberg, J. (2023). Instead of language: Confusion. Sigmund Freud/Sándor Ferenczi. In: R. Soreanu, J. Staberg, & J. Willner (eds), *Ferenczi Dialogues: On Trauma and Catastrophe* (pp. 23–71). Leuven: Leuven University Press.

Index